THE WHICH? GUIDE TO
MANAGING BACK TROUBLE

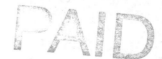

About the author

Dr Harry Brown is a full-time general practitioner based in the north of England. He has written extensively on medical topics in national newspapers and magazines. He is married with one son.

THE WHICH? GUIDE TO MANAGING BACK TROUBLE

Dr HARRY BROWN

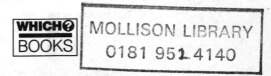

CONSUMERS' ASSOCIATION

Which? Books are commissioned and researched by
Consumers' Association, and published by
Which? Ltd, 2 Marylebone Road, London NW1 4DF

Distributed by The Penguin Group:
Penguin Books Ltd, 27 Wrights Lane, London W8 5TZ

Based on *Understanding Back Trouble* (Consumers' Association): text revised and
new material written by Dr Harry Brown

The author and publishers would like to thank Ann Holgarth and Gerry
Thomas of the National Back Pain Association, Claire Brown and Ami Sevi for
commenting on parts of the typescript.

First edition July 1996
Copyright ©1996 Which? Ltd

British Library Cataloguing-in-Publication Data
A catalogue record for this book is available from the British Library

ISBN 0 85202 603 X

For a full list of Which? books, please write to
Which? Books, Castlemead, Gascoyne Way, Hertford X, SG14 1LH.

Cover design by Ridgeway Associates
Cover photograph by Adrian Hobbs
Typographic design by Paul Saunders

Typeset by Business Color Print, Welshpool, Powys, Wales
Printed and bound in Great Britain by Clays Ltd, St Ives plc, Bungay, Suffolk

CONTENTS

Throughout the book the names of relevant organisations are marked with an asterisk (*). Their addresses and telephone numbers can be found in the address section at the back of the book.

FOREWORD

BACK pain can be devastating when it strikes. The pain may be intense and incapacitating and to the sufferer there may seem to be no relief, let alone a cure. But there is hope. The National Back Pain Association, committed as it is to education, research and support, is delighted to have been involved so fully with *The Which? Guide to Managing Back Trouble*. This informative book offers plenty of food for thought, explaining the many treatments for both short- and long-term relief that are currently available. It also acts as a reminder that prevention is better than cure; this means looking after your back, keeping it healthy with regular exercise and using it correctly. It is never too late to change your posture, diet, exercise régime and the way you live your life. Let this book show you how.

Gerry Thomas
Director, National Back Pain Association

CHAPTER 1

INTRODUCTION

BACK pain is a common scourge of humanity – at least in developed countries. There can be few westerners who do not experience it, if only for a short while, at some time in their lives. There is no telling when it will strike because it will not necessarily be preceded by injury; it may be brought on by moderate physical exertion, poor or abnormal posture or by nothing specific.

No one can ignore back pain when it does strike, usually in the lower back, although it can be anywhere along the length of the spine. It can manifest itself as a 'crick' in the neck, a sharp pain between the shoulder blades, a cramp in the back of the waist or a deep ache across the hips, arms or legs. Often it can make it difficult, even impossible, to maintain some or all of the commonest human postures: sitting, standing and lying down. It can vary from a feeling of discomfort to one of the most intense kinds of pain known and can lead to a few days off work or even, very occasionally, prolonged disablement.

Back pain is not an illness but a symptom. It indicates a malfunction of the spine or its supporting musculature but says nothing about the causes; muscle strain, a trapped nerve and spondylitis are just three of the many possibilities. Not all back pain derives from the spine: the symptoms may be due to gynaecological problems, for example, or some type of kidney disease.

Even though most backache is a passing problem, early episodes of pain should not be ignored. The first two or three may last a few hours, days or weeks, and while they last, the sufferer can usually think of nothing else. Once the pain is over, however, it is soon forgotten. Most people, in fact, recover quite quickly, even without treatment. These attacks do tend to recur, and there may be a pattern, perhaps with each successive one lasting longer, and eventually the pain may be permanent. It is therefore wise to establish the cause of even moderate attacks of back pain in the hope of preventing recurrences.

Attacks of back pain can strike out of the blue, seemingly without any unusual stress or strain; they may, nevertheless, be the culmination of years of unwitting misuse or minor incidents in which small aches and pains have been disregarded. Some aerobics enthusiasts exercise through sensations of soreness, perhaps 'going for the burn' (that is, deliberately exercising until it hurts). It is unclear why some people who do these things are afflicted and others are spared. One reason may well be a hereditary factor, leading to a tendency towards structural weakness. Very tall or very stout people seem to be more at risk than others. However, just as some people worry compulsively, yet do not suffer from stomach ulcers, or smoke heavily without getting lung cancer, so there are people who court disaster by lifting heavy weights awkwardly, stooping over their work, sitting slumped in badly designed seating or being overweight – yet are never bothered by back or neck pain.

Nothing to show for it

Sufferers may have the additional problem of convincing others that they are really in pain. The cause of their complaint is not obvious, there is no visible abnormality and no objective way of verifying it. When a bone is broken and the limb is put in plaster, everyone knows why you are housebound for a while. With bronchitis and a course of antibiotics, people will accept that you are really ill. However, if you have back or neck pain, everyone will agree that you may need a few days' rest, but that may be all. Employers are sometimes intolerant of lost work time because they believe back pain is a 'skiver's charter' for casual absence or for the avoidance of certain tasks. On the other hand, some people with a highly developed sense of responsibility to work may be reluctant to take adequate time off. Many doctors would consider this attitude to be foolhardy, while some would recommend a speedy return to work as part of the philosophy of confronting pain rather than giving in to it.

The scale of the problem

Backache has reached almost epidemic proportions and is one of the commonest disabilities that an adult can face; a staggering 10 per cent of the adult population in Britain (if asked) would admit to having had a back problem that had restricted their activities during the past month. Illness through back trouble has had a major effect on Britain's economic performance. Estimates of work-time lost vary widely depending on what is being measured. One study, based on 1993 figures for Britain, claimed that 150 million working days were lost during that year. However, these figures were calculated based only on the working population and those eligible for welfare benefits, and did not take into account, for example, elderly people. The total cost to Britain in terms of treatment, lost production costs and welfare benefits (NHS expenditure on it is thought to be in the region of £500 million a year) could be well in excess of £5 billion a year.

It is thought that between three and seven million people consult their family doctor every year for backache, but this represents only the tip of the iceberg as there are many other people who do not visit their doctor. Although there are variations in the figures quoted by different surveys, the message is the same: backache is a major problem. The medical response, however, can be fragmented. GPs are likely to have had inadequate training to deal with it so they compete with a number of alternative and complementary practitioners. A wide range of options for secondary care is also available as a number of different specialists have an interest in backache; the sufferer may be referred to an orthopaedic surgeon, a rheumatologist, a neurosurgeon, a general physician or even a gynaecologist. In addition, patients might be sent to pain clinics, physiotherapists or occupational therapists, and occasionally psychiatrists have been involved. Unfortunately, however, it is the availability of local resources that often dictates who treats those who have back trouble.

The problem of knowledge

One of the difficulties about curing back pain is that diagnosis is problematic: a great number of possible causes may manifest themselves as back pain. It is also unclear why pain persists without structural causes. There is a tendency to attribute most back pain to the minority of causes that are understood. In addition to this, most forms of backache get better spontaneously, so it is difficult to know whether a particular cure has worked or if the back has simply healed by itself. Most experts, therefore, point to these successes as proof that their theories are the correct ones.

Improvements in the prevention and treatment of back trouble can happen only with an increase in knowledge. As a first step to finding out how not to misuse your back, it is worth getting to know how it is constructed and some of the ways in which it can be damaged.

CHAPTER **2**

STRUCTURES OF THE BACK

THE spine has three main functions:

- it is the main support of the whole skeleton
- it protects the vital and vulnerable spinal cord
- it provides attachment points for muscles.

The bones of the spine

The spine is composed of 26 bones; 24 of these are separate vertebrae stacked on top of each other to form a column. They are graduated in size so that the column is narrowest at the top, where the skull is balanced, and widest at the base, where it is balanced on the bony pelvis.

The spine is divided into five regions. Starting at the top, the first seven bones are cervical (neck) vertebrae. Next come the 12 thoracic (chest) vertebrae, each of them attached to a rib on each side, and the five lumbar vertebrae. Below them lies the sacrum, a curved wedge-shaped bone, which fits between the two hip bones of the pelvis; it consists of five sacral vertebrae fused together. A vestigial tail, the coccyx, composed of four tiny coccygeal vertebrae fused together, forms the thin end of the wedge.

A straight back?
The spinal column is not, as one might suppose, straight like a pillar; it has four curves. The cervical vertebrae curve forward and so do the lumbar ones (producing the hollow of the back).

11

The spine

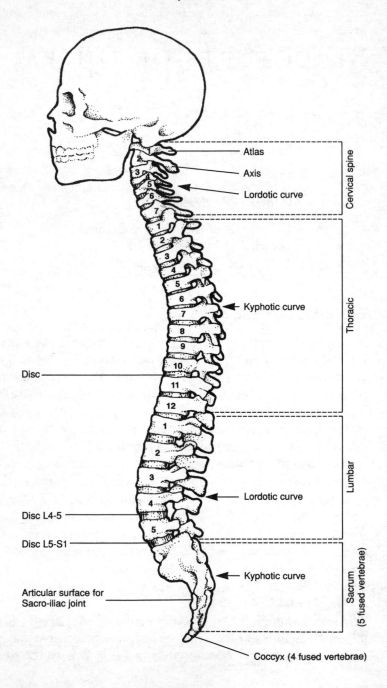

The medical name for such a forward curve is lordosis. The thoracic vertebrae curve backwards, medically called a kyphosis, making a hollow for the chest; the sacrum, together with the coccyx, also makes a backward curve. These natural curves make the spine more efficient at absorbing shocks and stresses.

The vertebrae

No two vertebrae are identical in shape or size but all have a roughly similar outline. Except for the first two cervical vertebrae on which the head swivels and tilts, each vertebra has a solid block called the vertebral body, facing towards the front of the trunk. The rest of the vertebra is called the neural arch and points towards the back. The arch is made up of several bony protrusions: two struts called pedicles jut out directly from the body. From these project a pair of sideways-pointing protrusions called the transverse processes. There are two more pairs of protrusions: the superior articular processes point upwards, the inferior articular processes point downwards.

These processes have oval, smooth cartilage-covered areas, called facets, which meet the corresponding surfaces above and below to form joints, called apophyseal joints or facet joints. Each vertebra is joined to the one above and the one below: each inferior articular process forms a joint with the superior process of the vertebra below it, and so on down the line. Like many other joints in the body, these vertebral joints are enclosed in capsules lined with a moist membrane called the synovium, which is lubricated with synovial fluid.

At the back of the neural arch is a protrusion called the spinous process. The bony layers between it and the rest of the arch, one on each side, are called laminae. The spinous processes are the knobs you can feel when you run your fingers down someone's spine.

The whole series of arches, stacked on top of each other, form a bony channel, down which passes the spinal cord, continuing from the base of the brain to the level of the first lumbar vertebra.

Intervertebral discs

The vertebral bodies are the weight-carrying parts of the vertebrae. They are separated by intervertebral discs, of which

Lumbar vertebra

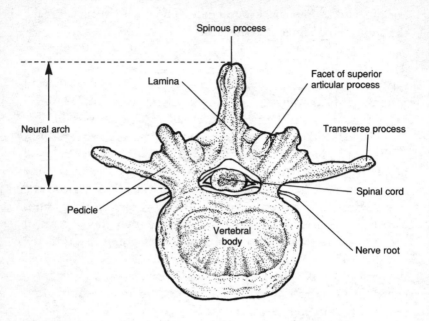

Spinous process

Lamina

Facet of superior articular process

Neural arch

Transverse process

Spinal cord

Pedicle

Vertebral body

Nerve root

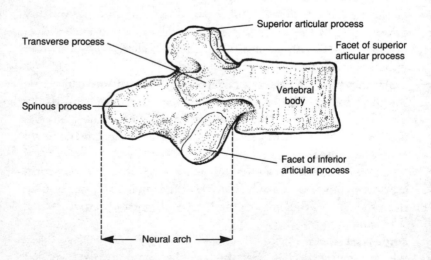

Superior articular process

Transverse process

Facet of superior articular process

Vertebral body

Spinous process

Facet of inferior articular process

Neural arch

SIDE VIEW

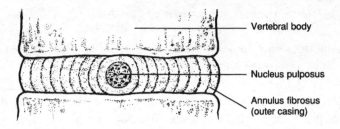

Vertebral body

Nucleus pulposus

Annulus fibrosus
(outer casing)

Disc when person is standing relaxed, with no loading

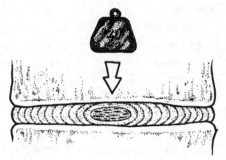

Disc when person is standing up carrying a heavy load

there are 23 – one between every adjoining pair of vertebral bodies. In normal use these discs are very efficient shock-absorbers; without them every step and movement would jar. The disc is a very tough structure: inside a strong fibrous casing (annulus fibrosus) there is a pulpy gelatinous substance (nucleus pulposus), soft yet firm and reinforced with strands of fibre. The disc has no blood, very little nerve supply and consists mostly of water. During daily activity, the pressures on the spine force some fluid from the discs into the vertebral bodies. This is reabsorbed by the discs during relaxation, so people actually become slightly shorter in the course of the day and taller during the night. As people grow older, the discs lose some of their fluid content permanently and become thinner.

The spine and movement
Altogether there are 149 joints in the spine. As well as those which link the vertebrae to each other, there are those which link the spine to other structures. For instance, the first cervical

vertebra is joined to the part of the skull called the occiput, and the sacrum is joined to the parts of the hip-bones known as the ilia, forming the two sacroiliac joints. The ribs are joined to the transverse processes of the thoracic vertebrae.

The bony basin of the pelvis holds and protects many vital soft structures in the abdomen, such as the intestines and the female reproductive organs. Being articulated with the hip joints, it transfers weight down the legs to the feet. The tilt of the pelvis is an important factor for the balance of the spine.

The individual shapes of the vertebrae govern the direction of their movements, permitting certain movements and not others. For example, the first cervical vertebra (called the atlas), allows the head to nod backwards and forwards and to tilt sideways. The second (called the axis) has a knob which fits into a socket through the atlas into the base of the skull; it allows the head to rotate, that is to turn to the left and right.

The thoracic vertebrae also allow backward, forward and sideways movement, and most of them also permit rotation, but only to a limited extent, because they are anchored to the rib cage. The lumbar vertebrae permit backward, forward and sideways movement only.

Ligaments

Wherever two bones form a joint, the two ends are bound together by fibrous bands or fibrous sheets. These are called ligaments and are very strong, mostly inelastic but with some 'give'. The fibres of each ligament are aligned along the lines of force occurring at that joint and control movement by allowing it only in a certain direction.

The ligaments of the vertebral column are of various types. The main ones are the longitudinal ligaments: long bands which run down the length of the spinal column, in front of, behind and to the sides of it. Other ones connect the process of adjacent vertebrae or connect the spine to other structures, such as the pelvis and the rib cage. The ligamentum flavum (yellow ligament) lines the back of the spinal canal, connecting the laminae of the arches; it is more elastic than other ligaments in the spine.

Three vertebrae of the lumbar spine

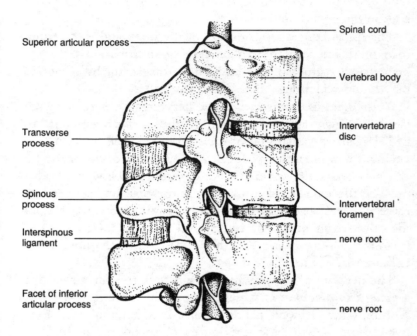

Superior articular process

Spinal cord

Vertebral body

Transverse process

Intervertebral disc

Spinous process

Intervertebral foramen

Interspinous ligament

nerve root

Facet of inferior articular process

nerve root

An intervertebral foramen is formed by the gap between the pedicles of immediately adjacent vertebrae

The spinal canal

This is the conduit through which the spinal cord passes. It is formed by the backs of the vertebral bodies and the vertebral arches and protects the spinal cord. The cord is surrounded by cerebro-spinal fluid and encased in the dural tube which is made up of three tubular membranes, one inside the other. The dural tube descends all the way to the sacrum, though the spinal cord ends in the upper lumbar region.

The spinal cord is an extension of the brain and is the trunk road of the nervous system, conveying information from the brain to all regions of the body and back again, by means of nerve roots which branch out from it.

At the level of each vertebra, the nerve roots emerge through chinks, known as intervertebral foramina, between adjacent pedicles, one on each side of each vertebra. Each nerve root is enclosed in a dural sleeve. From all these pairs of nerve roots a vast network of nerves branch out throughout the whole body.

Since the spinal cord stops short at the first lumbar vertebra, there is a sheaf of pairs of nerve roots passing downwards from the lower segments of the spinal cord to reach their respective foramina. This sheaf is called the cauda equina, the horse's tail, because that is what it looks like.

The network of nerves which originate in the nerve roots has a pattern of distribution which is much the same for everyone, with only minor individual deviations. It is therefore possible to trace a pain sensation in any part of the body, caused by a compressed nerve root, back to its point of origin in the spine. For example, a pain in the big toe that is caused by a compressed nerve must originate in the last two lumbar vertebrae or the upper part of the sacrum – nowhere else in the spine.

The spinal cord is not easily injured, except through fracture or dislocation of the spine or when the cord is penetrated by sharp instruments, bullets or shrapnel. In normal circumstances the spinal canal and its contents are protected from injury by bone, ligaments and muscle.

The spinal canal changes its length with spinal movement. When you bend sideways, it becomes longer on one side than the other. On bending forwards and flexing the spine, the whole canal lengthens, more so behind than in front. The change in length in the cervical and lumbar regions may be as much as 25 per cent, and the contents of the spinal canal adapt accordingly. When the spine is bent back and arched, the intervertebral discs tend to bulge forwards and the ligaments at the back of the spinal canal slacken.

In the course of vertebral movements, the gaps between each pair of vertebrae (the intervertebral foramina) open and close, as the neighbouring vertebral arches move closer together or separate, and the nerve roots move inside the foramina.

Muscles

Muscles are the fleshy part of the body and consist of long, thin fibres, bound together in bundles by connective tissue, and supplied with blood and nerves. What is remarkable about these fibres is that they can become shorter in response to a stimulus. The shortening is caused by protein filaments inside the cells which pull against each other; on relaxation, the muscles are pulled back into their original position, by gravity or by the action of other muscles. Sometimes the cells are unable to relax their hold – this involuntary contraction of a muscle is called a spasm and may be caused by pain.

There are, roughly speaking, two types of muscle: the involuntary and the voluntary. The heart and the hollow organs (digestive system, uterus, blood vessels, etc.) are of the first sort. They work without conscious control while life lasts; you do not need to instruct your heart to beat. The voluntary muscles are mostly under conscious control, so that it is for you to decide to move your limbs, for example; but you do not, of course, have to plan the movements of each muscle. When you decide to bend your knees, for instance, reflex actions determine the different movements of the several different relevant muscles, and you neither know, nor need to know, which ones they are.

The voluntary muscles also respond to various stimuli through reflex actions: when you touch a hot stove, messages racing along the nerves will jerk away you hand faster than thought.

Because they can be controlled, the voluntary muscles can be trained to work more efficiently. With suitable training, the nervous system learns how to recruit muscle fibres more rapidly and more precisely, and the muscles themselves become stronger and bigger and more capable of clearing away the waste products of their activity, so that they can continue working for longer. If they are not exercised, they waste away quickly.

The action of a muscle is to develop tension between two points on the skeleton, so as to draw them together or prevent them from being pulled apart, or control the rate at which they are being pulled apart. Without muscular control, the spine is much less stable, as in an unconscious person.

The muscles which control the spine are those of the back and neck and the abdominal muscles.

The muscles of the back

There are several layers of back muscles, their shape being different in each layer. No muscle crosses the mid-line demarcated by the vertebral column; for every muscle on one side of the back there is a matching one on the other side. Their points of attachment to the spine are the transverse and spinous processes of the vertebrae.

The largest back muscles are those in the topmost layer. They are triangular, extending in diagonal sheets across either side of the back, and they attach the spinous processes of the backbone to the shoulder blade and shoulder joints. These muscles hold the whole body steady when you are using your arms and legs to lift heavy weights.

The deeper layers are long, strap-shaped muscles extending vertically along the vertebral column. Most of them originate at a small area on the back of the pelvis, fanning out to attach themselves to various ribs as well as to vertebrae, and up to the head. This 'railway junction' on the pelvis is a common site of low back pain, which in some cases is the result of inflammation of these muscle origins.

At the deepest layers, the muscles are short and thick, extending only from one vertebra to the next, or its two or three neighbours, and keeping these bones aligned with each other; but they will stay aligned only if the muscles on either side are equally strong. If these small muscles go into spasm on one side only, at a particular level, the total posture is affected.

The abdominal muscles

These share the task of keeping the spine upright by exerting a pull down the front of the trunk that counterbalances that exerted by the back muscles. They also help the spine to bend by pulling the front of the rib cage closer to the pelvis.

Abdominal muscles also control twisting actions between the shoulders and the pelvis – no golfer could do without them – and they are used when pushing and for holding the posture when leaning backwards. When the body is bent sideways, they share the work with the back muscles on that side.

A muscle called psoas (from the Greek for loin) passes from the lumbar vertebral bodies, round the pelvis and over each hip-joint to the upper end of each thigh-bone. It contracts when you sit up from lying down. When it is active it pulls on the lumbar vertebrae, compressing the discs.

There is also an indirect mechanism by which the abdominal muscles support the spine. When a weight is being lifted, these muscles, in conjunction with the back muscles and the other muscles forming the abdominal cavity, tighten automatically. This increases the pressure inside the cavity, making it loadbearing (in the same way that inflating a balloon makes it able to support a weight), and as the compressed abdomen presses against the spine, it absorbs some of the load on the spine and helps the back to straighten up.

Weight-lifters deliberately increase their intra-abdominal pressure by wearing a special belt. For ordinary people it is enough to keep the abdominal muscles in good condition through simple exercises and keeping fit: this is very important for preventing backache.

What happens when you bend

When you start to lean forwards, the muscles of the back become active and tensed in order to counter the effects of gravity on the upper half of the body that is now forward of the hips, so that the trunk is cantilevered from the pelvis. There is a compensatory movement of the hips backwards to maintain the line of gravity within the base of support. On further bending, however, as the hands pass the level of the knees, the back muscles stop working and the strain is taken by the ligaments. The restraint on the

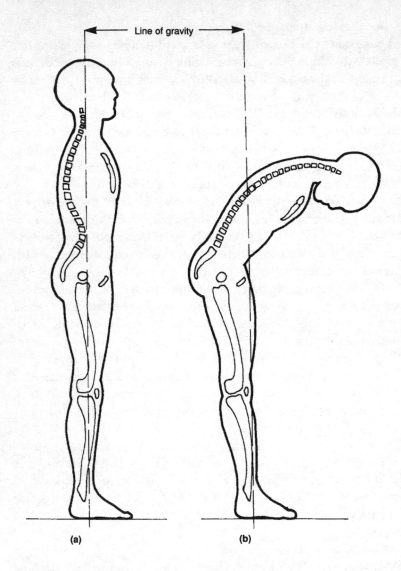

Line of gravity

(a)   (b)

(a) Line of gravity through the erect body. The disc spaces are approximately even in width from front to back

(b) When you bend forward, the discs are narrower at the front than at the back, and the length of the spinal canal between the cervical and lumbar regions can increase by up to 25%

(Note that in flexing the torso we move our legs backwards so that the pelvis is behind the line of gravity through the erect body; otherwise the weight of the torso would cause us to fall forwards.)

spine by either muscles or ligaments impose a force on it which compresses the vertebral bodies and discs. The muscles of the hip, thigh and back are strongly active when holding the trunk in the forward position and have to become even more active to bring the body upright again. The muscles do not resume their work until the hips are again at right angles.

Tendons and fascia

The muscles in the arms and legs are attached to the bones by means of tendons (sinews), which are tough, fibrous elongations of the muscle fibres. The muscles attached to the vertebrae are not always connected by tendons; in some places very tough, thin sheets of connective tissue, called fascia, connect the muscles to the vertebrae. A big band of fascia runs down the neck, becoming rectangular across the nape. There is another big, rectangular sheet of fascia at waist level. When the muscles are working strongly, the fascia and tendons take the strain at the point where they are attached to the bone.

CHAPTER 3

How the damage is done

THE various structures of the human back together form a complex piece of engineering. The backbone at one end is balanced on a tilting pelvis, and the other holds up a heavy head; at the same time it provides support for the movement of the arms and legs.

The skeletal system forms a mechanism which, although not properly ossified, is structurally complete at birth; it goes into full operation whenever a baby learns to stand and walk upright. The bones consolidate their shape during the teenage years and, under ideal conditions, should work perfectly for a lifetime. In practice, as we know, it is often otherwise. There are a great many ways in which the balance of the mechanism can be disturbed. Sometimes the damage is done in an instant, as the result of a single violent incident. At other times it is cumulative, the conclusion of a long series of small stresses. It has been thought that parts of the back, like those of any domestic appliance, may simply wear out through constant use. But there is no very good evidence for this: the resilience of most of the human body tends to belie such notions.

Stress on the spine

The spine can never be at rest while life lasts because the thoracic vertebrae, which are attached to the rib cage, move with every breath, straightening as you breathe in and flexing forward as you breathe out.

The spine plays a part in the movements of most other parts of the body. Moving the head in relation to the chest causes movement in the cervical and upper thoracic vertebrae; moving the arms also moves the thoracic spine; the lumbar spine is involved in movements of the upper part of the trunk in relation to the pelvis, and in moving the legs.

The spine and gravity

The vertical force exerted on the human body by gravity varies according to the position the body assumes. Gravity is least stressful in the lying-down position, and the stress is well distributed in moving on all fours (which is one reason why back pain victims sometimes have to revert to crawling); but the erect stance of *Homo sapiens* is maintained in defiance of gravity, and the gravitational load exerted on the head, arms and upper trunk is taken mainly by the vertebral bodies and the intervertebral discs. (Back problems are, however, not exclusive to those who happen to stand erect. There is a popular misconception that if only we walked on all fours, we would have no back problems. But some animals undoubtedly do have back troubles: horses, dogs – especially dachshunds.)

The muscles, too, undergo gravitational stress, depending on the direction of movement. In bending, the downward movement of the trunk is helped by gravity, with the muscles and ligaments controlling and limiting the descent; in straightening up, the muscles must do all the work, against gravity, but once the upright position is achieved, they do not need to work very hard to maintain it.

The effects of movement

Any muscular activity and movement causes some increase in spinal stress. If you stand on the bathroom scales and watch the pointer while you raise your arms, you will see it move up. The force needed to lift the arms is passed down your spine to your feet and (via the scales) to the floor. The same is true of every other activity – pushing, pulling, carrying, getting up, sitting down.

Body movements that are caused by outside forces also cause stress on the spine. Most forms of transport, from horses and bicycles to trains and buses, bounce and jolt the human frame; apart from jolts and jars, most people occasionally stumble or fall.

The force of all such vibrations is imparted to and resisted by the spine, but in most cases it suffers no serious injury, because of its capacity for absorbing shocks. It converts the energy into movement by going with the impact instead of resisting it and alters the quality of the applied force, so that it is less likely to cause injury.

The function of converting force into movement is a vital one. Unless some of the applied energy can be quickly converted into movement, it will break bones or cause other injury. In young and supple people, much more movement can be produced than in someone who is old and stiff, and they can therefore take more punishment than elderly people. As well as being more mobile, the structures in a young spine can bend or change shape more readily in response to loads and muscular tension. This is why young people are better than old people at 'taking' forces and reducing them.

Spinal functions also include a safety mechanism: namely, protective backache or pain. Pain is information and mainly of value in giving warning of postural stress. It is not so effective at preventing injury caused when something proves too heavy to lift or will not move because it is, unexpectedly, stuck – then the pain may come too late.

Damage to the discs

Intervertebral discs are not easily injured. The gel-like nucleus of the disc allows it to change shape, rather like a cushion that is sat on, in response to pressures that are exerted on it. The tightly-woven fibres of the outer casing, the annulus, are very strong and moderately elastic so that, like a cushion cover, it is able to accommodate, without tearing, most changes in the shape of its contents. However, although strong, it is not invulnerable. It may tear if subjected to a twisting action, that is, any movement in which the vertebrae above and below the disc are made to rotate in opposite directions. This sort of injury can be caused by an untoward movement in the course of vigorous exercise, for instance, or through lifting a heavy object awkwardly. It is most likely to happen when the trunk is bent forward: in this position the lumbar facet joints are less effective at preventing rotation.

Damage to an intervertebral disc

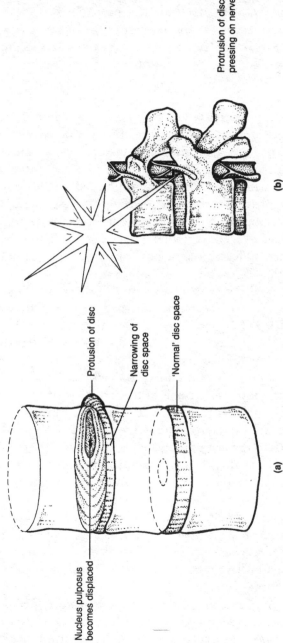

Nucleus pulposus
becomes displaced

Protusion of disc

Narrowing of
disc space

'Normal' disc space

(a)

Protrusion of disc
pressing on nerve root

(b)

(a) When an intervertebral disc is damaged by injury, disease or faulty posture, the fibres of annulus fibrosus become weakened and allow the disc to protrude at the edge

(b) If the protrusion encroaches upon the spinal canal or an intervertebral foramen it could press upon a nerve root and cause severe pain

When the tear is very severe, the pulpy nucleus of the disc is forced out by the pressure of the vertebrae above the tear (like toothpaste squeezed out of a tube), and protrudes out of the tear. Such an injury is rare. If the outer casing does not tear, the nucleus will remain contained within the casing, but its pressure may cause the disc to bulge outwards.

Prolapsed disc

If the protrusion or the bulge does not press on any sensitive structures there are no symptoms because the disc has almost no nerve supply of its own. If the bulge presses against one of the ligaments which bind the spine together or against a nerve root, the pain can be intense. This condition, called a prolapsed disc, is what is popularly, but incorrectly, called a slipped disc. A disc cannot, in fact, slip out of place because its fibres are knitted into the bone of the adjacent vertebral bodies.

Any disc may suffer a prolapse but, for reasons that are not well understood, those most frequently affected are the last two in the lumbar spine – the one that lies between the fourth and fifth lumbar vertebrae (L4.L5) and the one between the fifth and the sacrum (L5.S1). One reason why discs at those sites become affected may be because those are the points of maximum movement for the lumbar spine.

The commonest direction for a prolapse is backwards and sideways. The symptoms arise from the irritation of the sensitive structures and the associated inflammation, similar to the inflammation following any injury. This develops over a day or so, and spreads to involve other tissues at the same vertebral level. It may cause back pain or sciatic pain (down the leg), depending on whether it affects the tissues of the spine or of the nerve root, or both.

Prolapsed discs resulting from violent injury are probably likeliest to occur in young people who are most apt to go in for strenuous games, 'working out', disco dancing, and so forth; young nurses also have a fairly high rate of disc injury through lifting and turning patients.

In middle-aged people, however, it is gradual degeneration of the casing of the disc, rather than violent exercise, that is the commonest cause of disc prolapse. The fibrous outer casing of the disc gradually weakens and grows stiffer, developing cracks through which the nucleus can leak out.

As a small compensation, disc prolapse becomes much less common once middle age is past and this, too, is due to degenerative changes. The nucleus, losing much of its moisture, shrinks considerably, and though it may spread out, it is less apt to leak out of the casing. However, this change brings its own problems, as the disc loses some of its shock-absorbing ability.

Damage to the bones

The vertebrae, like any other bones, can be fractured by a blow, accidental or deliberate: a car crash, a fall from a height or a bullet may chip one of the vertebrae or even detach a fragment. Too vigorous exercise may do the same: if a tendon attached to one of the transverse processes is overstretched it may come away, taking a piece of the bone with it. Violent, unskilled physical effort may also cause microscopic fractures in the cartilage covering the flat sides of the vertebral bodies.

Compression forces which are too powerful for the discs to absorb – for instance, the violent jolt of a leap from a height, as in a poor parachute landing – may cause a crush fracture of a vertebra, shattering the vertebral body or forcing it out of shape, or breaking off the transverse processes.

Spinal fractures are often, but not invariably, painful; they usually mend with rest. A crush fracture may displace part of a vertebra so as to produce a slight hump that can be seen and felt. Sometimes an X-ray discloses bone damage of which the owner of the spine was unaware, and which gave no trouble. However, the most serious fractures, those that damage the spinal cord, can cause paralysis below the site of the injury.

Spinal trauma
Spinal trauma is one of the most horrific forms of injury; when the spine is fractured, the spinal cord, which is the extension of the brain that lies at the centre of the vertebral column, can be damaged through bruising, haemorrhaging, lacerations and, at worst, it can be completely severed. Any paralysis below the level of the damage is likely to be permanent as the spinal cord cannot

recover. Situations that can cause spinal trauma are injuries resulting from, for example, a fall from a horse, diving accidents or collapsed rugby scrums.

The higher up the level of the injury, the greater degree of paralysis; transection of the spinal cord in the neck may affect the nerves that control breathing (the ability to breathe may be lost completely); if this happens the injured person must receive mouth-to-mouth resuscitation or artificial respiration immediately, otherwise he or she will die. Contact the **Spinal Injuries Association***** for counselling and information support.

Spondylolysis

A fracture or crack of the vertebral arch in the lower lumbar spine is called spondylolysis. It may happen either suddenly or gradually as the culmination of a series of repeated strains (rather like a fatigue fracture in metal), or as a result of a congenital defect. It often causes no symptoms and a person may have it all his or her life without knowing.

Spondylolisthesis

This is a condition in which a vertebra slips forward out of alignment with the part of the spine below it. It commonly arises in the fourth or the fifth lumbar vertebra, so that all the rest of the spine moves forward out of line with the sacrum. The usual cause is a defect or crack of the neural arch (spondylolysis), which causes the facet joints of the articular processes, which normally hold the vertebrae in line, to loosen their hold.

Much less commonly, the slippage may be in a backward direction; it is then called retrolisthesis.

The causes of the trouble may come from a hereditary weakness of the neural arch: it seems to run in some families and some races, and is particularly common among Inuit. It may, however, arise from injury, such as a heavy fall on to the coccyx; or from constant stress, as in the case of athletes and gymnasts; or simple from wear and tear in middle age.

In spondylolisthesis the damage, unlike many vertebral fractures, does not heal spontaneously, perhaps because the lumbar spine has a natural forward curve.

There may be severe pain if deformation of the neural arch or the displacement of a vertebral body causes pressure on a nerve, or if the slippage damages the disc fibres and brings about a prolapse.

Cumulative damage

Most damage to the bones of the spine, however, is cumulative. The spine is a symmetrical structure and can be damaged by stress that is unequally distributed. When the vertebral bodies are continually made to bear uneven stresses by being loaded more heavily on one side than on the other, wear and tear causes irregular shaping of the bone material.

Scoliosis

This is the name of a sideways curvature of the vertebral column. It may be a congenital condition, the result of muscular weakness on one side of the spine, or the consequence of bone disease in childhood. Misalignment of the shoulders and hips, with one appearing higher than the other, is a common sign of scoliosis; women who have this problem cannot get their hemlines to hang straight.

If the condition is detected in childhood, when the bones are growing, it should not be ignored: treatment by splinting or bracing may be required to prevent the child from growing up badly deformed. If mild, the condition may get better without treatment. Spinal surgery may be advised in severe cases.

A less conspicuous type of scoliosis occurs in people who are born with one leg slightly shorter than the other. Quite often they do not walk with a limp, having become used to compensating for the inequality by curving the spine slightly towards the longer leg: in this way they keep the trunk level.

When the vertebral column bends sideways, the vertebrae automatically rotate slightly to accommodate the posture; this is unlikely to cause any trouble in the short term. However, a scoliotic spine is more prone to injury than a normal one because the curvature makes it harder for the vertebrae to rearrange themselves as demanded by all the activities of daily life. They may therefore lock or jam in one position. In the long term, they wear down more on one side than on the other, because the stresses on them are unequal, with resulting strain on the neighbouring joints and muscles, perhaps causing pain.

Another type of scoliosis is temporary and occurs in people suffering from a prolapsed disc or some other painful back problem. Their normal posture being painful, they instinctively adjust the position of the vertebrae to achieve a more comfortable position. This may bring its own problems because the spine is then unbalanced, but the scoliosis should disappear when the pain does. Contact the **Scoliosis Association UK**★ for information about congenital problems.

Damage to the joints and ligaments

The spine is organised so precisely that it is hardly possible to damage any one of its components without affecting all the rest, even though the effect of this may not become apparent for a long time.

Anything that alters the shape or position of the vertebrae causes additional stress on the facet joints which help to keep the vertebrae in place, and they, in turn, then exert more stress on the muscles and ligaments.

When all the joints of the spine are fully mobile, the sum of all the little movements that they are able to perform amounts to a wide range of activity – all that anyone should ever need. But if some of these joints should become stiff – something that one might be unaware of at the time – the other joints find it more difficult to carry out their normal range of movements. This, in turn, places the adjoining muscles at a disadvantage, causing them to go into spasm, which then puts stress on the work of the other muscle groups in the region.

Moreover, many people go in for daily activities which require the spine to move in ways that are anatomically unwise. Many so-called keep-fit exercises also demand movements which the spine is not constructed to perform, and which are stressful to the joints.

Whiplash injury is a good example of damage to a ligament that can cause serious and possibly long-lasting problems. It is commonly associated with car accidents, especially if a vehicle is shunted from behind, when the head can be jerked violently backwards and forwards. If the car stops suddenly the head is thrown forward and is only stopped from any further movement by the chest. In the recoil backwards, the neck can be overextended. This violent motion can damage and tear the ligaments in the neck and cause bleeding between the injured ligaments and the neck vertebrae. There may well be no symptoms for some hours after the accident, and it is unlikely that anything untoward will appear on the X-ray. The symptoms that occur later may be pain and stiffness and reduced movement in the neck.

There are different ideas about the treatment of whiplash, especially regarding the use of a neck collar. A soft supporting neck collar can be useful in the few days following injury but it should not be worn for more than a fortnight; over-use will result in the neck becoming chronically stiff. Physiotherapy and the sensible use of painkillers are other helpful treatments.

At the lower end of the spine, the pelvis is joined to the sacrum by the sacroiliac joints, reinforced by strong ligaments, which may, however, be damaged by a sudden jolt: by sitting down very hard, or by violent exercise that involves a twisting motion. A more common reason for trouble in this area is reserved for expectant mothers. Towards the end of pregnancy, hormonal action softens these ligaments in order to allow easier passage for the baby's head through the pelvic ring, and this makes the sacroiliac joints prone to injury. Once the baby is born, the ligaments tighten again over a period of several months.

However, if there is additional strain when the joint is loosened or if there are frequent pregnancies, the ligaments joining the two bones may never quite recover their original immobility.

Misaligned joints

The facet joints that unite each vertebra to its immediate neighbours may be jerked out of alignment by severe sudden stress, such as a twisting movement: this is called subluxation. A still more violent movement may pull the bones even further apart so that the joint becomes unstable; this is called dislocation. It is uncommon unless there is severe force. Subluxation may also be the result of growing older. The intervertebral discs flatten out as they lose their moisture, so that the spine becomes shorter and the ligaments which support it become slack. This may allow some play in the facet joints, with a greater chance of misalignment.

Both types of injury, subluxation and dislocation, are more likely to occur when the body is bent over and the joints are already undergoing tension.

In either case, there is some tearing of the ligaments that bind the facets together, and which are part of the synovial capsule enclosing the joint. There may be some internal bleeding; the irritated capsule becomes inflamed and swollen and there is pain.

Stress on the ligaments

The ligaments in an adult have very little elasticity. They can be strained, that is, over-stretched by violent action, usually at their points of attachment to the bone. They can also tear, usually in the direction in which their fibres are weakest. Torn ligaments heal rather slowly (more slowly than bone).

Ligaments do not contain blood vessels; any bleeding which occurs when a ligament is torn comes from the surrounding tissues. This results in the formation of fibrin, protein fibres which form new tissue to mend the damage. Often this causes scar tissue to form along the line of the mend (rather like excess glue along the cracks in repaired china), and this may adhere to the surrounding tissues, hampering the movement of the ligament. Further strain may wrench and tear these adhesions, causing more inflammation and pain.

Joints at risk

The little facet joints at the side of the spine take more mechanical strain from unequal stresses on the spine than the main intervertebral joint itself. The subsequent inflammation is a common cause of low back pain, particularly the type that gets worse with exercise or as the day goes on.

The facet joints in the lower lumbar spine have the function of preventing the vertebrae from rotating, and so are especially vulnerable to damage from twisting movements, but joint injuries may occur anywhere along the spine.

At the upper end, strain on the cervical vertebrae can send the neck muscles into spasm, producing a 'stiff neck' (called torticollis, or wry-neck). This usually gets better in a short time when the spasm decontracts.

Damage to the muscles and tendons

The muscles which support the spine and control its movements are liable to injury by the same stresses that damage the vertebrae and joints. Muscular injury may be related to postural stress or to excessive or miscalculated effort.

An example is bending with a sudden jerking movement without allowing the back muscles to arrange themselves for co-ordinated effort. This can cause excessive strain to the muscles which have the job of controlling bending movements of the spine.

Any unaccustomed effort can injure a muscle; keep-fit and other exercises which do not begin with a warm-up period can result in aching muscles or even injury. People who rashly dig the whole garden after a winter's inactivity are likely to suffer for it.

Another way to do damage is to lift heavy or awkwardly placed loads, particularly if this involves bending or off-centre one-armed efforts, or sideways twisting.

Muscular spasm: the pain/spasm cycle
In most parts of the body, following injury or pain, the involuntary response of the surrounding muscles is to contract in a spasm, clasping the hurting part as in a vice. This prevents it from being used any further, and so protects it, but it also impedes the blood circulation. If the pain was caused by pressure on a nerve, the spasm reinforces the pressure, setting up a kind of vicious cycle. For the damage to be repaired and the function in the damaged part to be restored, the muscular spasm must first relax.

Muscles at risk
Each movement of a joint is a harmony of different muscle actions. Some muscles shorten to produce the movement. Other opposing muscles allow themselves to be lengthened to control

the movement, a third set of muscles is busy cancelling out unwanted associated movements to enhance the performance, and a fourth set of muscles is holding the body fixed and firm to provide a solid foundation on which movements can take place. If the muscles around some of the vertebrae were to jerk and tug in opposite directions, there would be pain and muscle spasm, causing these vertebrae to be pulled and twisted even more. Ligaments and tendons could be damaged, and the muscle tissue become inflamed. One example of such unbalanced action is twisting oneself out of a car seat while carrying a heavy bag, or manoeuvring an infant into a car seat in the rear of a two-door car.

It is important for the muscles to be trained and worked equally on both sides of the vertebral column. If an action uses mostly the muscles on one side, a deliberate effort should be made to follow that action with another that uses the muscles on the other side. For instance, when polishing, a spell of using the right arm should be followed by an equally long spell of using the left arm – or vice versa.

Asymmetrical stressing is particularly damaging in childhood, when the bones are growing; while symmetrical pressure encourages the bone to become dense and strong. Any weights that are carried should be evenly balanced on both sides of the body, with a straight back.

Injured muscles can be extremely painful, but as a rule they recover completely with no treatment other than rest. Healing may be total but where it is accompanied by shortening of the muscles, rendering the structures more vulnerable, some therapy gradual stretching – will help.

Muscle pain from postural stress

Most people at one time or another experience the discomfort of aching muscles caused by adopting an awkward posture. For instance, holding a book at arm's length is hard work on the shoulder muscles, not because the book is heavy, but because it is exerting a leverage at the end of the long arm, and this greatly magnifies its weight. In contrast, when that leverage is removed by simply letting the arm hang, the task is easy. Leaning forwards over a bench imposes the same kind of stress on the muscles of the back, for then the weight of the head and trunk is exerting leverage through the spine on the hips and lower back of up to four or five times as much as when the body is upright. If these postures are sustained, discomfort and pain may result. As a general principle, the more intense the muscle tension, the sooner the discomfort begins. It is therefore important to change postures frequently, to share the load of any task between all the muscles that may reasonably be harnessed to help and to take adequate rest breaks. A series of short routine actions can also cause muscle tension and postural fatigue if repeated too often, as in assembly-line work in a factory.

The bad design of some equipment and furniture used in work, both domestic and outside the house, readily causes muscular stress in the user. It is also true that many people let themselves in for unnecessary muscular ache, in the back and neck muscles and elsewhere, by adopting a bad posture: such as sitting slumped in a chair, or humped over a desk.

Pain in the back muscles caused by postural stress can generally be relieved by rest and/or change of position and postural retraining. In extreme cases, it may become chronic and require treatment. Also, when a neighbouring part of the spine is painful and inflamed. the back muscles may be held taut to guard against a painful movement, and this in turn may fatigue them and make them ache. The additional pain resulting from this tightening of the muscles can be a considerable component of the pain experienced. Consciously trying to relax can help; if not, treatment of the inflamed condition will be needed to relieve the soreness in the muscles.

Not all muscular pain is caused by postural stress. Anxiety and frustration can give rise to muscular tension. If the frustration has no outlet or the anxiety is not relieved, muscular pain can occur. Tension in the shoulders and neck can also produce headaches.

CHAPTER 4

AGEING AND DEGENERATIVE CHANGE

As we get older, our whole spine tends to become stiffer. Not only is the total range of movement reduced, but the tissues in the spine are stiffer and change shape less readily; this reduces their shock-absorbing capacity.

To some extent, degenerative change can produce similar effects locally in individual joints. A completely degenerated intervertebral joint – disc, ligaments and joint facets – is stiff, fibrous and narrow.

Degenerative change can start in the teens, but the likelihood of it increases with age. It differs from the ageing process, however, because while ageing affects the spine as a whole, degeneration generally begins in a single intervertebral segment. There may be advanced degenerative change in just one site, with apparently normal discs and joints above and below it.

Degeneration may begin in the disc itself or in the joints or ligaments – particularly the interspinous ligaments which join the vertebrae.

Degenerative change tends to begin much earlier in people who do heavy unskilled manual labour. It can also start early in people who go in for strenuous forms of exercise – but some experienced weightlifters show no more degenerative change than sedentary workers. It seems that violent exertions and unskilled efforts are most likely to cause minor damage to the cartilage between discs and vertebral bodies, or to the ligaments. If they are repeated often, there is a cumulative effect leading to degeneration, even though at the time each injury felt no worse than a momentary jarring. There is also some evidence that prolonged awkward posture may lead to such damage.

Degeneration does not necessarily lead to back pain. Plenty of people undergo degenerative changes, which show up on X-ray, without ever suffering from back pain.

Disc degeneration

A completely degenerated disc is much thinner than a normal one. On an X-ray, this shows up as a narrowing of the space between vertebral bodies, since the disc itself does not show on X-rays. As well as being flattened, it is stiff and fibrous; at this stage it is unlikely to cause back pain. When the degenerative process has reached this stage of stiffness, and the nucleus has dried out, there is much less risk of prolapse, and the system is stable.

It is in the earlier stages of degeneration that disc injuries and pain are more likely. The disc is much weaker than it was formerly, and much readier to bulge. It can therefore become the source of repeated back trouble. Mechanically, it can no longer restrain the shearing forces between the vertebral bodies as efficiently as it once did, and therefore the joints and ligaments may have to resist greater strains than they are designed for.

A sign of degenerative change is the appearance of small ruptures in the annulus fibrosus (the outer casing), and the pulpy nucleus tends to spread through these. It is at this stage that some people undergo a disc prolapse which can cause trouble.

Ligament degeneration

Ligaments also undergo degenerative changes. The interspinous ligaments often begin to degenerate in people whose spine has become so stiff that they can no longer bend forwards. The ligaments become narrower, and their structure can become disorganised by ruptures and cavities. They then become a likely source of pain and local tenderness. These changes can occur in one ligament or a series of ligaments involving various levels of the spine.

Degeneration also affects the ligamentum flavum (the more elastic ligament which lines the back of the spinal canal), particularly when the spine has become stiff, and the ligament is no longer stretched normally. It becomes more fibrous, loses its elasticity, and can become a source of pain.

Joint degeneration

When the spinal joints are subjected to abnormal wear and tear, such as repeated strains, the cartilage which lines the joint facets becomes thinner and more fibrous, and the articular processes tend to become thicker where they are attached to the capsule of the joint. This thickening reduces the space in the spinal canal and the intervertebral gaps. Degenerated facet joints can become the site of back pain, and of pain felt over the buttock and down the thigh.

Osteophytosis

This is not a degenerative condition in its own right but may be a secondary manifestation to a degenerative disease. It is the formation of osteophytes, bony growths or spurs, on bone, or fibrous tissue attached to bone. They are deposits of calcium, the material of bone; in the spine they form all round the edges of the flat sides of the vertebral bodies, and on the facet joints.

Osteophytosis is in fact a feature of osteoarthrosis (also called osteoarthritis), a degenerative disease of the joints. (It should not be confused with rheumatoid arthritis, which is an inflammatory joint condition.)

Although on X-ray osteophytes can look formidably hook-like, they usually cause trouble only if they happen to grow out into the chinks through which the nerve root pass, or into the spinal canal itself: if nerve tissue is compressed, this can be very painful. Such problems are most likely to arise in the lumbar region, where the cauda equina, with its bundle of nerves, emerges from the dural tube. Osteophytes can cause back trouble in people who have by nature a very narrow spinal canal.

Spinal stenosis

The condition of spinal stenosis can be a long-term result of both degeneration and osteoarthrosis. The spinal canal which contains the spinal cord can be narrowed by the processes of enlarged facet joints and the presence of bony osteophytes. This may be more likely if the spinal canal has always been small or if spondylolisthesis takes place. The net effect will be to decrease the diameter of the spinal canal, thereby exerting pressure on the nerve roots and spinal cord. The resulting symptoms include aching and numbness in the thighs and legs; in addition there may be pins and needles that radiate down the legs. The symptoms tend to occur only a few minutes after walking or standing erect and they are characteristically relieved by sitting or squatting. In other words, they are exacerbated by extending the spine and eased by flexion of the spine. Occasionally the symptoms can be similar to those caused by circulatory disturbances of the legs, and this can lead to diagnostic confusion.

X-rays of the spine may show spondylolisthesis or advanced disc degeneration with marked osteophytes. The width of the spinal canal can be measured from a plain X-ray but more precise information can be obtained from advanced diagnostic imaging techniques (see Chapter 8). Sensible measures to relieve symptoms include losing weight and taking advice on spinal posture to help reduce extension of the lumbar spine. If these measures fail, an operation may be required to relieve the pressure on the spinal cord.

CHAPTER 5

OTHER BACK PROBLEMS

THE kinds of back trouble that have been described so far derive from either some dysfunction of the spine, a congenital deformity, violent injury, or gradual deterioration with use and age.

There are, however, other kinds of back trouble. Some of them affect the spine mainly or solely; others affect various parts of the body, the spine being just one of them. A third category includes diseases which produce back pain without necessarily involving the spine.

Ankylosing spondylitis

This is a chronic inflammatory condition, or arthritis, pre-dominantly affecting spinal joints and tending to run in families. The hereditary risk of developing ankylosing spondylitis can be assessed to some extent as there is an association between the condition and a genetic marker called HLA B27. Most patients with ankylosing spondylitis will prove positive for carrying this marker. It affects men more than women, and symptoms often start when the person is young. It is a systemic disease, that is, it is not confined to the lumbar spine, and other parts of the body, for example, the eyes, may also be affected.

In ankylosing spondylitis, the same process of laying down calcium deposits which creates osteophytes may continue to the point of fusing together some vertebrae, so that the spine in that region becomes completely stiff.

It often starts in the lining of the sacroiliac joints and spreads gradually upwards to the other joints of the spine; it sometimes also spreads downwards into the hips and, more rarely, other leg joints. Over a period of time the inflammation may cause the ligaments of the joints to calcify, so that the joints become *ankylosed* (rigid) producing, in the worst cases, a spine locked permanently in a bowed posture. The ligaments joining the ribs to the spine may also harden, flattening the rib cage and making breathing difficult; this is one of the early symptoms. Others are pain and stiffness in the hip joints, which feel worst in the morning, as the condition is aggravated by lying still, and relieved by movement. Painkillers and anti-inflammatory drugs as prescribed by the doctor will help considerably. Exercise is invaluable, but it should be taught by a physiotherapist. Done regularly, it may help to keep the joints flexible and avoid severe deformity. Many patients take up squash, tennis, swimming and other sports and prefer this to the repetitive use of formal exercises over many years. Contact the **National Ankylosing Spondylitis Society★** for more information.

Arachnoiditis

This is an inflammation of the arachnoid mater, one of the three membranes making up the dural tube, which sheathes the spinal cord, and the dural sleeves, which sheathe the nerve roots. The inflammation causes the membrane to grow thicker and proliferate, particularly round the nerve roots, where they enter the dural sleeves. The nerves inside then become crowded and cannot move freely in and out of the sleeve. The result is back pain and also pain down the arms and/or legs, with tingling or pins and needles.

Arachnoiditis can be caused by some infection involving the cerebro-spinal system, such as meningitis, and can also occur as the aftermath of surgery on the spine, through the formation of scar tissue inside the dural sleeves. There is no effective treatment except symptomatic pain-relief.

Osteoporosis

This is a bone condition associated with growing old (although it can affect young people) and it may affect any bone, not just those of the back. It takes the form of loss of bone material (calcium and minerals), making the bones fracture more easily.

The spine tends to shrink in overall length, and the person becomes shorter. In advanced cases, the affected vertebrae may collapse in a series of crush fractures, so that the sufferer develops a curvature of the spine, becoming round-shouldered. The 'dowager's hump' seen in elderly women may be caused in this way.

Women at risk of developing osteoporosis are:

- Those who have an early menopause, perhaps before the age of 45
- Longstanding absence of periods (e.g. someone suffering from the eating disorder, anorexia nervosa)
- Family history of osteoporosis
- Prolonged bed rest
- Long-term, high-dose oral steroid therapy
- Heavy smokers.

Osteoporosis is common in post-menopausal women and women whose ovaries have been removed and can be, therefore, partly associated with sex hormones. In these cases, the condition responds dramatically to treatment with oestrogen-hormone replacement therapy.

Physically active people are less likely to develop osteoporosis as exercise is thought to have some protective function. Bone loss can be the result of prolonged immobility; this is one reason why doctors discourage patients from staying in bed longer than is absolutely necessary. Astronauts spending weeks and months in space beyond the reach of earth's gravitational pull also suffer bone loss.

The loss of bone is not in itself painful, but as the spine adapts to its new conformation pain may occur anywhere along it and in the joints between the spine and the ribs. Loss of spinal bone leading to crush fractures may cause trapping of pain-sensitive structures, such as nerve roots.

Osteoporosis has been described as the silent epidemic as there are often no symptoms until the bone density has fallen to such a precarious level that even the most minor trauma can result in a fracture. All bones can be affected but common sites, in addition to the spine, are hips and wrists. Minor falls or injuries can result in more serious injuries because the bones in these sites have become weak. It is helpful to identify those people who might have problems with osteoporosis so that something can be done in advance to try to prevent it. Plain X-rays give only limited information about bone loss so more sophisticated techniques are needed to measure bone density. Specialised scanning equipment can be used to measure it but unfortunately these facilities are not widely available in Britain.

Hormone replacement therapy is the most widely used treatment, but other therapies which may help osteoporosis sufferers do exist; some of these drug treatments are quite new and not yet totally established but, nevertheless, do offer some hope.

Paget's disease (osteitis deformans)

This is a bone disease of unknown origin, which may occur in any area. It usually starts in middle age and is rarely found before the age of 60. The bones thicken and become denser, but also softer, and tend to deform. In the spine, Paget's disease may cause pain through pressure on the nerve roots; painkillers may suffice.

Most sufferers do not need treatment as they either don't have any symptoms or, in some cases, don't even know that they have the disease. It is often picked up on an X-ray only as an incidental finding. If necessary, there are specialised treatments, which can be used if severe bone pain is not responding to normal painkillers; for example, potent drugs are now available which can control the increased rate of bone re-modelling.

Rheumatoid arthritis

This disease is predominately one of the limbs but it can affect any joints, including those in the spine. It is the commonest form of joint inflammatory disease and typically affects the joints symmetrically (e.g. both wrists or both hips), causing destruction and deformation of those affected. Primarily it is an inflammation of the synovium, which is the tissue that is wrapped around a joint. Fluid from that inflamed tissue can gather in the joints, making them swell. The cause remains partially obscure although we do know that there are abnormalities of the body's immune system.

Rheumatoid arthritis can occur in different patterns: in one, or many, areas suddenly, or slowly over a number of years. It often causes stiffness and aching in the smaller joints such as the ones in the hands, though any joint can be affected. Attacks tend to recur and finally may leave the joint quite damaged. Rheumatoid arthritis does not usually affect the spine at the start of the illness but it can affect the lumbar spine later on when the disease has been present for some time; more worryingly, it can affect the cervical spine, which is the essential life-sustaining structure that controls breathing.

Subluxation (partial or incomplete dislocation) of the upper cervical vertebrae is not an uncommon finding, particularly in long-standing rheumatoid arthritis. Although usually associated with no more than neck pain, in certain circumstances there can be problems. For example, if the neck is manipulated either by an osteopath, a chiropractor or an anaesthetist, sudden cord compression could occur; therefore always discuss your medical history fully with your practitioner before consenting to a treatment regime. This would cause similar problems to that of a spinal injury.

The treatment of rheumatoid arthritis involves using drugs both for pain relief and in an attempt to alter the natural history of the illness. In addition, expert help may be needed from rheumatologists, orthopaedic surgeons, physiotherapists and occupational therapists.

Other causes of back pain

The symptoms of backache are sometimes mimicked by other illnesses not connected with the spine. Blood tests are done in addition to X-rays to eliminate the possibility that one of these illnesses is responsible for a patient's problem. The most serious of them is a tumour on the spine, causing back pain by compressing a nerve. This is no more than a remote possibility: in the great majority of cases the back pain is in fact found to be due to some mechanical disturbance.

Everyone is familiar with the ache in the bones that goes with influenza; many other viral infections produce some degree of inflammation in the joints. Occasionally the pain may be severe in the lower back. In such cases, however, there are sure to be other symptoms such as high temperature or a sore throat; if the infection affects the digestive organs, there may be diarrhoea, nausea and loss of appetite. These symptoms indicate that the back pain, which is part of the infection, is likely to go when the infection goes.

Kidney stones and kidney infections may also produce lower back pain, but in this area, too, there are usually tell-tale symptoms, such as fever and pain on passing urine.

Women

Normal conditions, such as pregnancy and menstruation, can also give rise to back pain. In pregnancy, hormonal changes before childbirth cause ligaments to soften and slacken, and this can cause strain, particularly in the sacroiliac joints; the weight of the growing foetus also throws additional strain on the spine. Backache can be particularly uncomfortable in the last two to three months of pregnancy as the body prepares for giving birth. However, the backache does not always end once the baby is born as it takes a while for the body to resume its normal shape and function. In menstruation, period cramps are sometimes felt as referred pain in the structures of the back.

Stress

The mental stress caused by an attack of back pain can reinforce the effects of muscle spasm, and in turn be made worse by it, forming a vicious circle. Muscle spasm is a possible result of tension. A major problem is fear of pain, sometimes not so much fear of the pain itself as fear that it is really more serious than anyone supposes. The remedy then is to seek authoritative reassurance.

It also seems very probable that mental tension, stress and anxiety, unexpressed fears and worries can actually start off an attack of backache by increasing muscular tension throughout the body. (This also makes you more vulnerable to muscular and joint strain which may even lead to some sort of mechanical displacement.) There are cases in which stress-reducing measures, such as relaxation tapes, or perhaps counselling, rather than treatment are what are needed to relieve the pain.

CHAPTER 6

Where does it hurt?

THE body's central nervous system consists of the brain and the spinal cord, which is the brain's extension down the spinal canal. The nerve roots that pass in pairs out of the spinal cord at the level of each vertebra and at the sacrum, proliferate into an abundant network of nerves, some as long as one metre, reaching to distant parts of the body. They carry information about injury along the spinal cord to the brain, which acts as a control centre, where the information is interpreted in the form of a sensation of pain. The sensory nerves that bring it are able to convey information about the type of injury; thus, the pain of a blow is different from that of a pinprick.

Pain is not sensed in the injured tissues themselves: the experience of pain is registered in the brain. For pain to be felt, there must be, or have been, a nerve supply. Some structures of the body have little, or none: for instance, the nucleus of an intervertebral disc. If it is damaged, no pain will be felt unless part of the disc presses on one of the nerve roots, the dural tube or on a ligament. Therefore the absence of pain does not necessarily mean that there has been no injury.

There can be an interval, sometimes days, between injury and the sensation of pain. If you are concentrating hard on something else, you can often override the pain message. Sportsmen, in particular, often fail to realise that they have been hurt, until the game they are playing is over. A severe pain can mask a lesser one, rather like a strong radio signal which suppresses a weaker one. Thus it may not be until the more severe pain has responded to treatment that a secondary pain reveals the presence of a lesser injury.

Pain is both a mental and a physical event, and the extent to which it is found endurable depends largely on individual temperament. Some people give way rapidly and take to their bed, while others grimly remain at their posts, regardless of suffering. There is an intelligent compromise between these extremes: an awareness that pain is, in general, a warning of injury or risk of injury through misuse or malfunction, which should not be neglected.

Referred pain

It is common for pain to be felt in an area much larger than the site of the injury, in remote tissues, which apparently have nothing wrong with them. This is called referred pain; its mechanism is not well understood but it probably occurs because the perception of pain can be felt as being anywhere in the network supplied by a particular nerve root. Information about any part of that region of the body reaches the brain along the same neural route. That is why people are able to feel pain in 'phantom' limbs that have been amputated. The pain message from the nerves in the stump are interpreted as if coming from a whole limb.

Pain in the back

Any of the tissues of the spine can be a source of pain except for the discs and the cartilage of the facet joints which have no nerve supply.

If the pain arises in the more superficial muscles, it can be identified as coming from a particular spot. Pain from around the facet joints and ligaments is less easy to pinpoint; and if it arises as the effect of a ruptured disc, it is felt too diffusely to locate precisely.

When it is the nerve root that is irritated, pain can be felt anywhere in the region which that nerve supplies. Thus, pain from injury to the sacral or lumbar nerve roots may be felt in the low back or to one side, or, very often, down one leg on the same side as the nerve. Disturbance to cervical or upper thoracic nerve roots may produce similar symptoms in an arm. Pain from the waist region is often felt in a buttock or the groin. Similarly, pain originating in the ligaments and joints of the lumbar spine may be felt across the back of the hips, round the groin, across the buttocks, along the thigh to the knees or even further down the leg.

A sufferer's doctor or manipulative therapist should be helped to identify the level in the spine of the source of pain by an exact description of where the pain is felt and its nature.

Root involvement; nerve-root lesion

These are medical terms for the condition in which a nerve root is being irritated by being compressed or angulated so that its blood supply is restricted. As well as pain, there may be other symptoms; if the nerve is of the motor type, whose function is to stimulate muscles into activity, the affected muscle may become weak and have a reduced reflex response. It is seldom that all the nerves of a nerve root are damaged: as a rule, only a small proportion of them is affected.

Constant irritation of the nerve root in its dural sleeve may set up inflammation throughout the surrounding tissues, and this can cause adhesions to form between the walls of the spinal canal and the dural tube, which sheathes the spinal cord, and also in the intervertebral foramina, the facet joints of the vertebrae, and the surrounding ligaments. These adhesions prevent the nerve root from moving easily in and out through its foramen with the normal movements of the spine and limbs, and this may cause pain. If a disc prolapses backwards, the prolapse can, depending on the size of the spinal canal, involve the cauda equina itself. This is rare, but if it happens, the resulting back and leg pain, with numbness, weakness and disturbance of bowel and bladder function, creates a surgical emergency: seek medical aid without delay.

Other symptoms

Pain may be accompanied by other symptoms, such as a feeling of dullness or heaviness, or perhaps coldness or a tingling sensation. When a lumbar nerve root is irritated or compressed, there may be weakened muscles as well as pain; a loss of sensitivity in the skin of the leg and the foot; pins and needles; tingling, heaviness, constriction or cramp.

CHAPTER 7

WHEN THE PAIN STRIKES

AN attack of back pain can take several forms. It may occur as a sudden, acute pain at a particular site, and be so severe that you cannot move; it may begin as a dull ache that becomes more severe during the following 24 hours; it may appear as a less painful sensation of stiffness in the muscles down one side of the body.

Back pain may follow a bout of unaccustomed exertion, such as clearing a garden path after a snowfall or moving heavy furniture at spring cleaning. You may also bend down awkwardly or with a sudden jerk and feel that something has 'gone' in your back, but not experience really severe discomfort until the next morning, when inflammation will have built up in the damaged tissues. An attack may come on after a spell of mild, nagging backache which you had ignored in the hope that it would go away.

If you have had back trouble before, quite mild and accustomed exertion can cause it to recur; for example, reaching across the car from the driver's seat to open the passenger's door.

Immediate action

In the case of an acute attack of back pain, stop whatever you are doing, even if you are only sitting down.

Get to a bed, or some other level surface, and lie down. If you are locked in a stooped or sitting position and cannot straighten up, you may have to crawl, or, having reached the bed, you may have to roll gently and slowly on to it.

Lying down takes the stress off your spine, so there should be less pain after a while. If your muscles are in spasm, this will help them to relax. You can then try to straighten yourself gradually, moving your legs gently until your spine is straight, with its normal hollow in the small of the back. If you can achieve this, it may help to bring the attack to a speedier end.

If you have suffered an attack of back pain in the past and can tell that another is threatening, it may be wise to go and lie down straight away.

Which way to lie down?

The stress on the spine is least when you lie on your back, but this may not be the most comfortable (or, rather, least painful) position for you. There is no single 'correct' position, so lie on your side or stomach if this suits you better. The position you adopted during a previous attack may not be right for you now. (Lying on the floor, perhaps on a blanket or sleeping bag, is often more comfortable than a bed or sofa.)

You need not lie absolutely flat, but it is best to make do with only one pillow under your head. Use whatever pillows or cushions you need to relieve strain. If lying on your back, a small pillow or folded towel in the small of the back and/or two or three pillows under the knees may make you more comfortable.

If you choose to lie on your side, try putting a pillow between your knees to support the upper leg and to prevent its weight from dragging on the spine and twisting it. The shoulders should be kept in line with the hips. Do not let the pelvis fall forward while your shoulders sink back against a pillow at the head. This would cause a definite torsion (twisting) in the spine, and you might feel worse stiffness and worse pain after spending some time in this position. Hugging a pillow in your arms may help to keep you lying correctly.

If your pain is in the vertebrae of the neck, you need something to give your neck support. Specially shaped neck pillows (which look rather like horse-collars) are available in department stores, but if you do not have one, roll up or twist a face towel lengthways and wrap it round your neck. A soft pillow loosely tied in the centre and filling shaken down to the two ends also makes a useful neck support. The thin middle part should lie behind the neck so the 'wings' support the side of the head.

Sitting, not lying
If there is nowhere for you to lie down – or if you feel more comfortable sitting down – try to find a suitable chair. It should have a firm seat to support the pelvis evenly; a soft chair will allow the pelvis, together with the spine, to tilt sideways, causing uneven pressure and muscle spasm. The back rest should have a slight backward slope, with cushions between you and the back of the chair, so that you can recline; the pressure of your body weight will then be dispersed rather than taken by the vertebrae. Every part of the body should be supported so that the muscles can relax completely.

The height of the seat should be such that your feet can rest flat on the floor without strain, or else they should be supported by a footstool.

Coping with the pain

Take a painkiller. Simple painkillers are often quite effective. A good example is paracetemol, but there is a range of over-the-counter medicines to choose from. If you are confused with the bewildering array of painkillers on sale, talk to the pharmacist. Do not be afraid of taking the full dosage recommended on the packet, for two or even three days at regular intervals, if necessary, with or after food (or at least a drink of milk). Do not try to use alcohol as a painkiller – especially not in combination with painkilling drugs.

There are many commercial backache treatments on the market, and many people swear by various folk remedies, perhaps ones that have been handed down through families. Most of these 'cures' owe their reputation to the fact that, untreated or not, most back pain subsides in few days. Any remedy being taken at the time usually gets the credit. There is probably no harm in using such treatments if you feel that they are doing you good, so long as they do not have untoward side-effects.

Hot and cold
Many people get relief from applying heat to the site of the pain. An ordinary rubber hot-water bottle inside a cover or wrapped

in a towel is simple and effective, but make sure that it is not hotter than you can bear.

A hot bath may be comforting, but you may find getting into it excessively painful – and getting out again could be worse. If you do have a bath, it is easier to kneel in order to get out, rather than trying to stand from a sitting position. If there is a risk that you may get stuck, take your bath kneeling. From a safety point of view, it is a good idea for someone to be available to help, if necessary, while you are having a bath.

A gentle back rub can help to relieve back pain by encouraging muscles locked in spasm to relax, and by producing warmth through friction. Any willing member of your household can do it for you, making sure not to start with cold hands (the room should be warm, too). There is no advantage in using ointment or liniment, but no harm in doing so.

For those who can bear it, the application of cold can also be effective in relieving pain, by numbing its site. If you have no ice-bag, you can use a hot-water bottle or even a polythene bag filled with crushed ice-cubes, or a pack of frozen peas will do very well. Make sure there is a damp towel between the ice and the skin. This treatment, like the heat one, should be used only in moderation (and only if found effective). Ten to twenty minutes is usual, or up to half an hour, but you should be aware that ice can 'burn' if the application is too prolonged. Anyone with a heart condition should avoid this form of self-help.

Bed rest

Although it seems comfortable to rest the back as much as possible, the current thinking seems to be that bed rest should be kept to the shortest time possible, and early activity should be actively encouraged. The maximum period recommended is three days for acute back pain. If there is nerve-root pain, more bed rest may be required but at this point you are likely to be under medical supervision.

Calling your doctor?

When the pain first strikes it can be frightening, and your first impulse may be to call your GP. But if the pain is only in your back, there is no need to be precipitate – and certainly no need to get your doctor out of bed. The pain should become less acute in a day or two, and the whole episode will possibly last three or four days. If you do call your doctor right away, the chances are that he or she will tell you to take it easy, take painkillers and ring again in two or three days' time if the pain has not lessened.

But if you have any other signs and symptoms: numbness, pins and needles, tingling; if you pass water very frequently, or have trouble doing so; if you experience weakness, giddiness or nausea; if you have severe referred pain (that is, somewhere else, as well as in the back), then see your family doctor. Failing this, speak to him or her over the telephone first as advice can help to clarify the situation. There are no hard or fast rules about when to consult your doctor but if you are not sure, it is better to be safe than sorry.

Staying in bed

'Put a board under your mattress' is the piece of advice that the back pain victim hears from practically everybody. But this should be necessary only if your bed has a very soft base or an old, sagging mattress. There is no need to support a reasonably firm mattress. However, if you do need a bed board but have not got one, ask someone to drag your mattress on to the floor. Or simply do what many back sufferers do, sleep on a quilt or sleeping bag spread on the floor itself, using pillows, as already described, to relieve pressure and to keep your spine straight. When in acute pain, it is difficult to get down on to the floor and even harder to get up again; going via the kneeling position helps.

If you lie mostly on your back, you may find it most comfortable to support your legs, from the knees down, on a pile of cushions; or on a chair or a stool or pouffe if you are sleeping on the floor. In this position, the back is kept from arching by being pressed firmly against the mattress (or floor).

If you have managed to find a comfortable position, the tendency is to stay put, but you should try to vary it from time to time, to help circulation. Also, if you remain immobile because of back pain you may find yourself feeling stiff all over after a time. Changing position may call for some courage: do it slowly and gradually. Changing from a horizontal to a vertical position is what hurts most, so do not try to sit up. As for turning over in bed, you may find this easier to do if you bend your knees, bringing your heels up towards your buttocks, and, keeping your shoulder in line with your hips, let the knees fall to one side and use the weight of your legs to roll you over.

For getting out of bed, try this method: turn on your side, then edge over to the side of the bed, keeping your knees bent; then let your legs slide over the edge, acting as a counterweight as you push yourself upright with your arms. Have a chair at hand to lean on as you get to your feet.

In the end, you will probably work out for yourself, by painful trial and error, the method of getting out of bed that causes the least discomfort. Even so, try to limit the number of occasions of doing it, especially during the first day or so. Moderation in eating and drinking will limit the number of times you have to go to the lavatory; and you may not have much appetite in any case. Avoid alcohol, which may interact with the painkilling drugs you are taking; some people find that it makes the pain worse.

You may find yourself temporarily constipated, which may be the effect of taking some types of painkiller, or of immobility, or fear of the pain that getting out of bed causes. This is a temporary problem, and there is no need to worry or do anything about it.

Keeping moving

At this stage you cannot do much in the way of exercise, but try to move your legs at regular intervals. The longer you remain immobile, the longer it will take you to recover your strength and mobility.

Even when you are suffering severe pain and are frightened to move, there are bound to be some movements you can make without pain.

Start with these: try wriggling your toes, bending and circling your ankles, working the feet up and down, bending and extending the knees. Do this for a few minutes, every hour or so. If any movement causes you pain, avoid it and try to find another that does not. In between spells of leg movements, do some slow deep breathing.

A weight off your mind

It may not be easy for you to induce your tensed muscles to relax if at the same time you are brooding about the work and other obligations for which you are now temporarily disabled. A serene frame of mind may seem rather too much to expect from someone who is being racked by acute back pain, but relaxation involves both body and mind, so if you can find a way of relaxing your mental tension, the pain may affect you less.

The best thing to do is to accept the situation and abandon, as much as possible, feeling of guilt about neglected work, missed appointments and so on. You are a victim of *force majeure*: the matter is out of your hands for the time being. You will have to ask someone to do some telephoning for you, cancel engagements and arrange for other people to stand in for you at home and at work. Accept the need to rest and look after yourself for a few days. The more you can allow yourself to be philosophical about the situation, the more rapid recovery is likely to be. For a while the world will have to roll on its course without you. This advice is more easily than followed.

But don't become an invalid

Other people can affect your back pain. Some families enjoy making a fuss of an invalid and that may actually inhibit the natural desire to resume normal life. One danger of giving in to back pain for too long is that stiffness and weakness ensue.

Supporters of the 'pain confrontation' school of thought argue that there is no evidence that activity is harmful and that, contrary to common belief, it does not necessarily even aggravate the pain as long as specific activities which increase the load on the spine are avoided. Increased activity may promote bone and muscle strength and may increase endorphin (pain-reducing hormone) levels and reduce sensitivity to pain. They also claim that there is no evidence that early return to work increases the likelihood of future recurrences. These views are not universally accepted.

When the pain starts to go

Most episodes of acute back pain grows less severe within two or three days, when the sufferer can start to get up and about again.

On the first day this should be for only a couple of hours at a time, with spells of rest in between, increasing gradually on succeeding days.

Getting dressed may be difficult, especially putting on socks, shoes, tights and trousers, and it may be wisest to stay in dressing gown and slippers for the first day or so you are up. If you feel that you must get dressed, wear whatever is easiest to put on. A woman can choose a dress rather than trousers, and leave off tights. Slip-on shoes are preferable to lace-ups. A long-handled shoe horn can be a help.

If you must put on tights or trousers, put them on while lying on your back with your knees bent; but do not raise your hips to pull them right up, which could arch your spine – get off the bed and then do the pulling-up.

There is a gentle exercise that is worth trying when you are feeling less sore. If the pain is in the lower back, while standing put the palms of your hands on your hips, on the bony crests on either side of the pelvis, and holding it steady, sway your shoulders backwards beyond the level of your hips, thus extending the vertebral column. Do this slowly and gently, and stop at once if the pain increases.

If the pain is in the upper part of the back, interlock your fingers behind your head; press your elbows back in line with the shoulder joints, pulling the shoulder blades together. Press your head slowly and gently against the fingers, while pressing your hands forward and up, thus applying a mild traction force to the neck. Again, stop if the pain increases.

Do not drive a car, and take care, when you are a passenger, how you get into your seat. Bending at neck or waist may bring the pain on again. Get in slowly, preferably by standing with your back to the seat, then sitting down with your legs outside, and then slowly swivelling round while lifting your legs in, with your hands behind the thigh.

Until you are completely fit again, do your best to avoid lifting and carrying heavy weights. If you really must carry things, essential shopping, for instance, divide the load equally in two, one bag in each hand. Or you could try a back pack, which someone else would have to put on for you. Above all, make sure not to repeat the movement which brought on the attack, if you know which one it was; and in general, avoid twisting and bending movements.

If the pain does not go

If after a few days, perhaps from day three, the pain is as bad as ever then it is probably time to see the doctor. If you are unable to get to the surgery for whatever reason you may have to request a home visit. If possible, try and request the house call early in the morning so the doctor has time to organise his or her day to fit in the request for a home visit. The doctor may ask:

- about the nature of the pain – you should tell him or her whether it is a sharp, stabbing or burning pain, or a dull ache; whether you feel it at one side or radiating to other places, the arms or legs, for instance; whether you are having tingling sensations there, or a feeling of numbness;
- about the origin of the pain – tell him or her when and where you first felt it; whether any particular activity had brought it on; whether it started suddenly or developed gradually; whether there are any postures or movements which make it worse – or better;
- about the duration of the pain – tell him or her how long it is since it started; whether you have it all the time; whether it has got worse since the onset, or stayed the same; whether there are times during the day or night when you feel it more.
- about medication you are taking, in particular drugs that you have purchased over the counter. Otherwise, the doctor may give you a prescription for a drug that may interact with an over-the-counter medicine.

The doctor may not follow this pattern; listen carefully to the questions and be as precise as you can in your answers. He or she may also ask you about the kind of work you do – active or sedentary, domestic or outdoor – in order to assess the stresses that it may exert on your spine.

The physical examination
You will be asked to remove your outer clothes. The doctor will ask you to do a number of things to enable him or her to assess your problem.

While standing upright, you will be asked to bend, as well as you can, backwards, forwards and sideways, so that the doctor can see which of these movements causes you most discomfort. This gives him or her a clue as to which of the joints or muscles of the back may be involved.

As you lie prone (face downwards) on the couch, the doctor will palpate, that is, explore by finger pressure, the tender area of your back, as well as other areas where you may not have felt pain before, but which are now found to hurt when prodded. This is because when the source of the pain is a nerve root, the pain may be felt all along the nerve.

As you lie supine (on your back) on the couch, the doctor will raise each of your legs in turn, with the knee straight. This stretches the sciatic nerve, and he or she will want to see how far this can be done without aggravating the pain.

The doctor may try other movements to find out whether certain nerves are working properly. He or she will check whether there is any loss of sensation in any part of the body, and whether your reflexes are normal.

In most cases, back pain is due to a dysfunction of the spine. However, there may be other causes, which the doctor is bound to consider: for instance, kidney disease or a peptic ulcer. So the doctor will probably examine your abdomen as well. In women, low backache from any cause may be worse before a menstrual period.

The doctor may give you painkillers, possibly by injection, and also tablets to take at home. In addition, you may also be prescribed a tranquilliser, not to stop you worrying, but because of the beneficial effect that a relaxed mood has on muscles in spasm. Tell the doctor if you happen to know that any of these remedies upsets you.

The doctor may also suggest treatment from other practitioners. Examples may include a physiotherapist and possibly a chiropractor or an osteopath. You may not always need your doctor's permission to see these practitioners but it might be useful discussing it with your GP. Access to osteopaths and chiropractors is usually not available on the NHS, but this trend may be changing. Very often you will have to pay to see them privately, but you will have the advantage that it is likely you will be seen pretty quickly. Physiotherapy is available both privately and on the NHS, but many areas in Britain have long NHS waiting lists to see them. Finally, your GP may send you to a hospital out-patient clinic for a specialist opinion.

CHAPTER 8

SPECIALIST EXAMINATION

IF your back trouble is not better after a few weeks, or, having got
better, keeps recurring, or your GP thinks there could be some
uncommon reason for your trouble, you may be advised to see a
specialist. Usually this means going to a hospital as an out-patient
(or being admitted as an in-patient for investigation and treatment)
to attend a consultant's clinic in the orthopaedic, rheumatology or
neurology department. The out-patient appointment may be for a
date weeks or even months ahead, though if your case is
considered urgent, you may be seen more quickly.

In the letter of referral, your GP will give the specialist a
history of your trouble, mentioning his or her own conclusions
from the examination and any tests carried out, such as X-rays.

The specialist's aim will be twofold: to exclude the possibility
that the pain is caused by disease in some other organ, and to find
out its origin and cause. The questions, the examination and any
suggested further investigations will all be directed to this
purpose, their scope depending on whether this is your first spell
of back trouble or a recurrent problem which has not yielded to
treatment.

The specialist will want to know about your previous medical
history, operations, severe injuries or prolonged illnesses, and
whether you are currently having treatment for any other
condition.

When the tests and investigations have been completed, the
specialist may be in a position to tell you whether there is any
serious disease. If you are not reassured on this point, do not
hesitate to ask questions.

Questions and answers

The first thing the specialist will ask is where the pain and other symptoms are, and how far they extend. Try to point them out as clearly as possible and be prepared to go into considerable detail, if asked. The specialist will want to know how long ago the trouble began; what you were doing when it started (or just before); what the symptoms were like to start with, and how they have changed since – in other words, whether you are between attacks, in continuous pain or getting better or worse.

If by the time you see the specialist your back is better, say so, as he or she will be used to this and will not think that his or her time has been wasted. The specialist's job is to get you completely well, and to prevent further trouble.

You should tell the specialist what makes the pain better, and what makes it worse – for example, bending, sitting, walking and so forth – and the effect the pain has on your usual activities. Tell him or her about your state of mind, too. Mention if you are under any strain in your work, home, relationships or other personal factors in case it has any bearing on your back pain. The severity and unpredictable nature of the pain and the disruption it is bound to have caused to your daily life may be affecting you emotionally.

It may be difficult to describe symptoms other than pain, such as heaviness, dullness, tightness, numbness and weakness. Numbness, for example, means different things to different people. Some use it in a general way to describe a sensation that a leg, for instance, has 'gone to sleep'. But it may also mean, more precisely, that the skin itself has lost all sensation and that you could scald it without feeling pain. Weakness, for instance, could describe feeling limp because of pain, or else being forced to drag your toes along because you cannot bend up your ankle. Analyse the feeling or pain carefully, explain it as descriptively as you can and try to make sure that the doctor understands what you are trying to describe. It is important for you, the patient, to tell the doctor what you feel, not what you think you ought to feel. Spontaneity is your greatest asset; leave the analysis to the doctor. Honesty is important: do not minimise or overstate your pain.

It is useful to be able to give information about any previous back trouble before the current attack. But when it is a long and complex story, it may be difficult to know how much to tell your doctor. On the whole, unless asked directly, it is better to avoid recounting in detail what has been said to you by various doctors, surgeons, chiropractors and physiotherapists you may have seen in the past. Doctors like to make their own diagnosis and it does not really help to give them other people's. The important thing is where the pain was and whether you had to go to bed or could continue at work; how many times you have had the pain since and whether the pain then, and subsequently, was like it is now; what investigations were made (if you know); whether you have had any treatment and, if so, what helped and what made it worse.

Going to a specialist can be an intimidating occasion. You may feel more confident if you jot down some notes beforehand, with dates, of your case history, so that you do not return home wishing you had mentioned all sorts of things you forgot at the time; it may also be helpful to note down any questions you may have about treatment options.

Physical examination

Be prepared to strip down to (bra and) pants with socks or tights off. The spine will have to be examined, and the examination is bound to hurt a bit because the pain is the focus of interest. Be as accurate as you can about what you feel while the doctor is examining you.

The order and extent of the doctor's examination may vary, but it usually begins by an inspection of the posture of your spine as this can be affected both by your present symptoms and by some deformity.

The range of movements you can make and the way you make them are looked at while you bend forwards, sideways and backwards; some hospitals have a special device for measuring this. The doctor moves your neck, arms and legs to test for signs of increased tension in the nerve roots, and also tests muscle strength in the back, abdomen, arms and legs.

Your spine is felt for signs of tenderness, muscle spasm or deformity. The sensitivity of the skin on the arms and hands or the foot, leg, thigh and buttock is checked by touch and pin-pricks. Your reflexes are tested at the elbow, wrist, ankle, knee and sole of the foot.

X-rays

You will almost certainly be sent to the X-ray department, either there and then or at a later appointment, to have X-rays (radiographs) taken of your spine. X-rays are two-dimensional pictures and are the result of a beam of X-rays passing through a three-dimensional image and irradiating a photographic film placed behind the image being visualised. The resulting film is usually viewed directly as a negative. If you are a woman of child-bearing age, mention to the radiographer if there is any possibility (no matter how remote) that you could be pregnant or are planning to be pregnant. Don't be offended if the radiographer asks this particular question as there is a good reason for doing so: an X-ray of the spinal area, particularly the lumbar spine, may irradiate the pelvis and could damage a growing embryo. Unless there are compelling clinical reasons for going ahead with the X-ray, if there is even a vague possibility of pregnancy it is better not to have one. This should be discussed with the person who has requested the X-ray.

Standard X-rays of the lumbar spine involve a dose of radiation about 120 times that of a standard chest X-ray. Patients are often very keen to have an immediate X-ray of their lumbar spine, and a refusal or hesitancy on the part of the doctor could be considered as an unsympathetic response. However, X-rays are not usually required in the initial management of backache in patients between ages of say 20 and 55 years. X-rays of the lumbar spine should be undertaken when there is a strong possibility of a serious problem. The yield of positive significant findings is pretty low; in fact it has been estimated that in adults under the age of 50, the pick-up rate of an unexpected finding can be as low as 1 in 2,500.

The X-rays are seen by the consultant, and may also be seen by the radiologist – a doctor specialising in X-ray diagnosis.

X-rays can reveal a fractured or cracked vertebra, or show the presence of degenerative changes in the vertebrae, such as the formation of osteophytes, or bone thickening, as well as signs of abnormalities such as misalignment of vertebrae, deformities and potential mechanical weaknesses.

X-rays can, however, be deceptive and show up an abnormality which causes the person no pain or, where a person is obviously in great pain, the X-rays may reveal nothing. The doctor may well not find anything abnormal, even though the patient may be suffering from acute disc prolapse or serious muscular injury because discs, muscles, ligaments and other 'soft' tissues are not radio-opaque: they do not show up on X-rays, or perhaps only very faintly. If the space occupied by a disc is seen to be reduced, it suggests that the disc has been flattened, but this does not necessarily indicate a prolapse.

Further tests

Depending on what has been learned so far, and on your symptoms, further tests may be carried out. In most cases, however, it is unlikely that they will have to be done; at any rate, not all of them.

Myelography

This is a method of making the dural tube show up in X-rays, by injecting a contrast medium – a radio-opaque liquid – into the cerebro-spinal fluid around the spinal cord. This done under local anaesthesia, by lumbar puncture: the needle is inserted through the skin of the back between a pair of vertebrae at the appropriate level.

Using an image-intensifying screen, the radiologist can see whether the spinal canal is abnormally narrow and whether anything is obstructing it – such as the bulge of a prolapsed disc or a degenerated joint. These show up as an indentation on the dural tube, or an obliteration of part of the dural root sleeve. In rare cases, back pain may be caused by a tumour on the spinal cord, and this, too, would be shown up by myelography. As a matter of routine, a sample of the cerebro-spinal fluid is taken for laboratory testing.

The lumbar puncture is done while you lie on a table that can be raised to the vertical, so that the radiologist can observe the movement of the contrast medium in the dural tube as you are tilted up and down. The table may also tilt sideways, or the apparatus rotate in relation to the table, so that the radiologist can view the spine from different angles. He or she will probably take still radiographs to record the significant findings. Most of the time, however, the radiologist will be studying the picture on a television monitor which you may be able to see, too.

When the myelography is finished, you may be sent to a ward, with instructions to rest quietly for up to 24 hours, and could be warned of the possibility of an adverse reaction to the dye or a severe headache as after-effects. Myelography is, to say the least, uncomfortable, but its use is waning nowadays because of greater availability of less invasive investigations such as CT scanning and MRI scans (see below).

Discography

This is a similar procedure, used for making discs visible on X-rays, and may show up prolapse bulges that do not show up on myelograms. The contrast medium is injected into the centre of discs, usually the three lowest lumbar discs. Only a small quantity of contrast medium is used, and the patient does not have to be tipped about. In a healthy disc, the medium stays discretely in the middle, but in a degenerated one it spreads out and may show the extent and direction of any prolapse. Apart from visualising the disc, the increase of pressure within it caused by the injection of the contrast medium may reproduce the patient's symptoms. This would confirm the diagnosis that the disc problem is a significant cause of the patient's symptoms.

CAT (or CT) scanning

CT (Computed Tomography) scanning is a further development of X-ray techniques. If X-rays are taken at different angles and from different view points, a computer can take this information and produce a picture that is relatively easy to understand. In essence, it can produce a picture of a slice of the body, showing structures inaccessible to a plain X-ray, thereby giving information about the spine and spinal column. The procedure takes a little longer than a normal X-ray, but it is not particularly unpleasant. The technique is sensitive enough to show up disc bulges and degeneration without any injection of contrast medium, though it can be combined with a myelogram.

Ultrasound scanning

This painless technique works rather like radar: by means of a microphone-like probe, which is passed over the back, inaudible ultrasound waves are directed at the spine, and the echoes which are bounced back are picked up by the probe. They are used to build up a picture of the spine on a monitor screen; one use of ultrasound is to measure the width of the spinal canal.

Magnetic resonance imaging (MR or MRI)

MRI is a technique that has rapidly gained acceptance as a powerful tool to image inaccessible structures such as the spine. It does not use X-rays but requires the patient to lie within a magnetic field. Short bursts of radiofrequency pulsations are applied to the patient, and hydrogen nuclei within the human body absorb this stimulus. When the applied radiofrequency stimulus is withdrawn, the hydrogen nuclei emit a signal which can be translated into pictures. MRI is now becoming the most popular investigation in the evaluation of low back pain and is fast replacing myelography. However, because it is relatively new (hence the technology is expensive) it may not be widely available. The cost of a new machine is about £1 million, and often a new building is required to house the machine. There are also significant annual running costs.

A scan involves the patient lying on a table with most of his or her body lying within the circular tunnel of magnetic coil. The patient must lie very still, and very overweight patients may not fit in the magnet. It is also possible that heart pacemakers may malfunction in a strong magnetic field, and patients with possible mobile metal objects inside their body, for example, surgical clips, may also be at risk. Many people also cannot tolerate lying still in such an enclosed space. Despite these drawbacks, MR scanning produces high-quality and extremely informative pictures of vital and otherwise inaccessible structures.

Electromyography (EMG)

This is done in some hospitals if damage to the nerve root is suspected. The functioning of the nerves that supply muscles is tested by using an apparatus for amplifying and recording the electrical activity produced in the muscles. A fine needle electrode is inserted into the muscles of the legs, and sometimes those of the back as well; this is usually not very painful – no more so than an ordinary injection – and leaves no side-effects.

The doctor may, in addition, do other tests to measure the speed with which nerves conduct the impulses in response to stimulation.

Blood tests
A blood sample may be taken, by means of a hypodermic syringe, from a vein in the arm, and sent to the laboratory for tests, in order to obtain more general medical information, particularly about the possibility of inflammatory joint disease, anaemia, viral infection or cancer.

Radioisotope scanning
Radioactive isotopes can be used to tag biological substances which will home in on such areas as bone. These tagged compounds are injected into the circulation, usually intravenously, and will find their way to their target tissue. Effectively, the radioisotope has a piggy-back ride to the area that is going to be studied. The target can then be scanned by special apparatus to pick up radioactivity, which can then be translated into useful pictures of, for example, the spine. Patients are naturally concerned about exposure to radioactivity, although, as a one-off event, the exposure is not excessive.

The tests
Although a bewildering array of tests is available, don't get too concerned about their technical aspects. Sometimes the choice of test may be dictated not by clinical need, but by availability. Large teaching hospitals may have the latest technology available, and smaller, more peripheral, units may have fewer facilities both in terms of equipment and personnel. However, not everybody with back trouble needs such sophisticated imaging. If you do need tests, a plain X-ray, and perhaps simple blood tests – facilities that are universally available in Britain – should be more than sufficient for many people. Only the potential candidates for surgery and those for whom a serious disease is suspected may have multiple investigations that require detailed imaging. However, if you are going for a test, don't be shy about asking why you are having this particular one and what difference this test will make to the management of your problem.

CHAPTER 9

TREATMENT

OVER the centuries, victims of back pain have submitted to a vast variety of treatments. The bizarre nature of some of these testifies to the sufferers' desperation: they were willing to try anything, even, it is said, having a tame bear tread on their back. In spite of great advances in medical science generally, these unorthodox treatments – except, perhaps, the bear – are still in with a chance.

Back pain therapy presents special problems as it is often difficult to diagnose the cause of an attack of back pain accurately. Damage to the structures of the back does not, as a rule, show on the surface, many injuries do not show up on X-ray, and even in-depth specialist investigations may not reveal anything obviously amiss.

Moreover, very often back pain is out of proportion to the problem causing it; although the pain is severe and disabling, the structural damage may be minor, and one accepted view is that it will heal, given time, with or without treatment. Another school of thought, however, considers this to be shortsighted and holds that correct treatment by a qualified therapist will expedite recovery and may help to break down scar tissue, the presence of which can produce long-term problems.

Whatever treatment is given it will certainly get the credit for the recovery. However, the next time it is tried, it may not work, either because it is valueless, or because the problem is not the same.

The information gleaned from each case may be of only limited use in the next one, and the treatment of back pain has had to be largely empirical. The fact that diagnoses are often less than accurate makes the choice of therapy problematic, and specific therapies which exist for one condition are sometimes applied erroneously to another. There is no scientific body of knowledge which allows a doctor or any other practitioner to state with certainty that a particular treatment will cure the trouble.

The rationale of advising rest, and particularly bed rest, is based on the clinical observation that lying down may relieve pain. This actually applies to a diagnosis of disc prolapse: intradiscal pressure is lowest in the lying position. However, disc prolapse constitutes only a small percentage of all low back pain, and treatment for disc prolapse cannot necessarily be applied to all low back pain. The time-honoured belief that bed rest is the first line of treatment for acute attacks of back pain is therefore undermined.

It is now conventional practice to limit bed rest as much as possible and promote exercise and rehabilitation. There is strong evidence against staying in bed for more than one to three days for acute back pain, although nerve-root pain, perhaps, may require between one and two weeks.

Basically, however, the treatment which is currently offered by most doctors starts with conservative methods.

Conservative treatment

The most obvious way of coping with back pain is avoiding the postures and movements that cause it, or make it worse. It is based on the supposition that, where there is no serious disease, the problem will diminish if what aggravates it is removed. Exercise is encouraged from the earliest onset of backache, obviously within the limits of the disability. The type of exercise is not important, but walking and swimming, in particular, could be helpful. If you decide to go swimming, make sure that someone is going to keep an eye on you; it might be worth mentioning to the lifeguard at the pool that you are having a problem with your back. These gentle pursuits place minimal strain on your back and most people can tolerate them. The amount and duration of the exercise routine should be gradually increased.

Physical treatment

Physical forms of treatment are generally safe and sometimes quite effective, especially for short-term use in an acute episode. The application of a cold pack, or even a packet of frozen peas, can bring relief; cold temperatures can decrease pain and muscle spasm during an acute episode as well as slowing nerve conduction. Athletes with soft-tissue injuries such as damage to the ankle often resort to this technique. Heat is another good form of physical therapy. In general terms, heat should be used for chronic problems and cold for acute situations. However, there are no hard and fast rules, and this maxim does not hold for everyone. The use of hot and cold should be reversed if you do not respond to or are made worse by either treatment; the correct one can be found only through trial and error.

Painkillers

Painkillers such as paracetamol and codeine have been used for many years in the treatment of backache. These are available, under different brand names in various combinations, for sale without a prescription at the local pharmacy. Often it is worth talking to the pharmacist about which preparation is suitable for you and your symptoms; always say if you are taking any other medication as this may have a bearing on the advice. The so-called non-steroidal anti-inflammatory drugs (NSAIDs) are also helpful in treating backache. Some are available on prescription whilst others can be bought over the counter. Ibuprofen is a popular example which is available both with and without a prescription. Side-effects of the NSAIDs are often associated with the gut, mainly causing indigestion and possibly even stomach ulcers. Other painkillers, such as the ones chemically related to codeine, can cause constipation which may make the symptoms of low back trouble worse; it might be sensible to increase the amount of fibre in the diet to overcome this potential problem.

Muscle relaxants

As the name suggests, muscle relaxants decrease the muscle-spasm which is secondary to backache. The drugs act on the brain to help reduce the muscle tension and in some people the use of such drugs, often in combination with painkillers, can be very effective, but because they act in the brain, their side-effects stem from their effect on the nervous system. Drowsiness, headaches and dizziness are commonly experienced side-effects. Some of these drugs may also impair concentration, so if you are driving a car or operating machinery, you might be advised to stop while taking them. Once the muscle spasm has settled down, these drugs should be stopped; they are not intended for long-term use (i.e. more than two weeks).

Anti-depressants

It may seem strange to suggest that someone with a physical condition should take anti-depressant medication. However, the mind is a powerful weapon and it is a well-known fact that sufferers from chronic pain, with or without depression, may benefit from the use of such medication. It possibly works by altering the way the brain perceives the pain messages it receives. In addition, sufferers of chronic pain (backache patients are no exception) can suffer from a depressive illness in addition to the back problem. Successful treatment of this complication can make the back-trouble symptoms a little more bearable.

Injection therapy

In some cases, pain can be relieved by injecting pain-relieving drugs directly into the area of the spine where the pain appears to be localised. It can be effective for treating 'trigger points' (fibrositis), which are small, very painful nodules of muscle, often in the buttocks, neck and shoulders; pressure on these points spreads the pain over a wide area.

Usually a corticosteroid drug is injected together with a local anaesthetic into the local area. The relief may not be immediate or long-lasting, and a number of injections may be required for the treatment to be effective. However, there are usually no adverse effects.

Epidural injections are used for pain that has not yielded to any other methods, the objective being to reduce swelling, inflammation and pain. The injection is given in the epidural space between the dural tube and the spinal canal, at the lower end of the spine. It consists of a corticosteroid drug mixed with a local anaesthetic. It numbs the tube and reduces inflammation caused by, for example, a prolapsed disc. The injection cannot cure the prolapse itself, but in most cases time is the best healer, and epidural injections, like other pain-relieving measures, make the period of waiting seem less interminable. It is an invasive procedure which requires a reasonable degree of technical skill and is usually carried out by an anaesthetist.

Complications are uncommon but headaches and very occasionally infection in the epidural space can occur. Steroids are noted for their potent anti-inflammatory effects, but they also have a reputation for causing side-effects, so an attempt is made to deposit them only at the site of the problem. The results of epidural injections vary and they do not work for everyone. However, if you are in a fair amount of pain and are advised to have an injection (either one or a course), it is worth trying

Much backache arises from the facet joints rather than from disc protrusion. Pain originating in facet joints can radiate down the leg and mimic sciatica. In some cases, injecting steroids and a local anaesthetic into the joint can stop the pain.

Chemonucleolysis (discolysis)

'Lysis' means dissolution. In chemonucleolysis, an enzyme called chymopapain is injected into the centre of the damaged disc nucleus. This enzyme is derived from the papaya (pawpaw) fruit, which is also used as a meat tenderiser. It has the effect of dissolving the more complex proteins in the nucleus and in the prolapsed part of the disc. Afterwards, the disc shrinks, becoming perceptibly narrower and stiffer. Because of this reduction in volume, the compression of the nerve is relaxed.

This method of treating a prolapsed disc is being offered in a few centres in Britain. It is a chemical alternative to disc surgery, and is used when time and rest have failed to reduce a disc protrusion which involves a sciatic nerve. It has much the same success rate as surgery, with different but no fewer risks, but it perhaps causes less discomfort and disablement during the recovery period compared with conventional surgery.

Chemonucleolysis is most successful in young people, and where the disc prolapse is fairly recent and has not had time to produce adhesions or cause nerve damage. It is least successful in the case of extruded disc-material having broken away completely, because the chymopapain cannot reach it.

How it is done
Chemonucleolysis is done under sedation or local anaesthesia; X-rays are used to place the needle accurately through the skin of the back. The specialist first injects some contrast medium into the disc to assess the damage, then, with the needle still in place, injects chymopapain. If the treatment is successful, the sciatic pain in the leg disappears, sometimes with dramatic rapidity; however, most patients have some backache for a week or two.

There is a considerable risk if the chymopapain is injected in the wrong place so the technique should be carried out only by experts. Even then, there is a small risk of an allergic reaction to chymopapain in patients who have become sensitised to it through eating tenderised meat, or who are allergic to papaya. Drugs are usually administered before treatment to minimise this risk.

Corsets and other supports

Various devices such as corsets, belts and collars exist for supporting the different levels of the spine. Even though these supports are restrictive and cumbersome, many people with back trouble are ready to put up with them for the sake of their benefits.

They work by slowing down all activity and restraining many small muscle movements, thereby helping muscular spasm to relax. Supports also prevent pain to some extent by stopping the wearer from making extreme movements. A corset can help with acute pain, in the early stages of recovery, and when an activity that might bring on pain cannot be avoided, for example, housework. However, it should not be considered as a long-term measure, as it has a tendency to weaken the muscles, and the wearer can easily become dependent on it. It is seldom necessary to continue with a corset for a long period; you should do so only if the specialist advises that it is necessary.

Lumbar corsets and belts encourage correct lifting and bending; as they restrict movement at the waist, the wearer is forced to lift things by bending, correctly, at the knees. They increase the intra-abdominal pressure which protects the spine in lifting actions by spreading the load, so that it bears less heavily on the lumbar joints.

Cervical collars are sometimes prescribed for neck injuries or for 'worn' neck vertebrae. They work in a similar way to corsets, giving support and preventing inappropriate movement. Like their lumbar counterparts, neck collars should be worn only as a short-term relief for an acute problem.

How to obtain a corset
The NHS supplies many different types of spinal and abdominal supports. Usually the consultant at the hospital or clinic will prescribe one, but in some areas the GP can do so, through the physiotherapy department. Corsets should be fitted properly by a physiotherapist or another professional health worker. They can be bought privately but are very expensive; ordering one by mail order may be unsatisfactory as the corset or belt may not fit.

A corset does not necessarily have to be worn all the time; ask for specific instructions about when and for how long you should wear it. Talcum powder on the skin underneath the corset reduces friction and may make wearing it more comfortable.

CHAPTER 10

PHYSIOTHERAPY

BACK pain frequently responds well to physiotherapy – the treatment by physical methods – as an alternative or adjunct to drugs or surgery. The methods include several different therapies: manipulative procedures, therapeutic movement or exercises and treatment with heat, cold and with electrical equipment. The aim is to help restore the function of the body and rehabilitate the patient; physiotherapy also includes advice and instruction on posture and daily activities.

The profession
Training for a physiotherapist in Britain is a three- or four-year course at one of the schools of physiotherapy attached to an academic institution, usually a university; the degree awarded is a BSc with, or without, honours. A student who passes the examinations qualifies for membership of the Chartered Society of Physiotherapy and therefore for state registration. Only state-registered physiotherapists can work within the NHS. Physiotherapists work in hospitals, local authority clinics, the community, special schools, industry and sports, and also private practice (and may visit a patient in his or her own home). It is not a closed profession (anyone can put up a plate and set up in practice as a physiotherapist), but only those who have passed the examinations recognised by the Chartered Society of Physiotherapy can put MCSP after their name; and those who are state-registered can put SRP. Contact the **Chartered Society of Physiotherapy**★ for more information.

Physiotherapy is an independent profession, and practitioners may accept people for treatment who have not been referred by doctors; this is more usual in private practice (in the NHS the vast majority of referrals are made through a doctor). The private physiotherapist may be able to give treatment more quickly than the NHS.

All health authorities have physiotherapy services. Patients are often referred to them by the consultant at the out-patient clinic they are attending. In many cases, however, physiotherapy clinics will accept patients by direct referral from GPs.

The doctor making the referral sends the necessary information about the patient and the condition to the physio-therapy clinic; this includes X-ray reports, with suggestions for the aims of the treatment, but the doctor leaves the choice of treatment to the physiotherapist's discretion. All physiotherapists assess patients and plan the treatment programme.

With all the changes in the NHS, it is possible that physio-therapy services may become more widely available in the community. For example, some general practices are now fund-holding and some of them have been able to use their funds to set up physiotherapy clinics in their surgeries. The result is that patients have the advantage of being treated locally and, possibly, having shorter waiting times.

Some specially trained physiotherapists are now seeing patients for initial assessments in hospital clinics, so patients do not need to see the specialist; hospital waiting-lists have been reduced as a result.

The treatment

Many people are unclear about what will happen during their first visit to a physiotherapist; he or she is a trained clinician, who will take a full, often extensive history. The assessment will also include an examination of your posture. The physiotherapist will then suggest a course of treatment that is appropriate to you and the current state of your back. This may differ from earlier treatments for what seems to be the same problem. A treatment regime for a bad back may include traction or gentle mobilisation possibly followed by manipulation. The treatment usually includes a regimen of exercises and instruction on how to lift and move safely.

What a patient does when not having treatment also plays an important role in recovery; the physiotherapist, therefore, will usually advise what he or she should do between treatments. Patients who hope and expect that the physiotherapist will work on them to get better are not pleased to discover that, instead, they are expected to participate actively.

Manipulative procedures

This is the term covering a very wide range of techniques from the very gentle to the more vigorous.

Soft-tissue techniques

The most familiar soft-tissue technique is massage whereby muscles, tendons and ligaments are mobilised by the therapist's hands and fingers in order to induce relaxation, increase local circulation and movement and relieve pain. Massage is usually used in conjunction with other procedures.

Regional mobilisation

For people with spinal problems, this is used to treat areas of stiffness and altered movement accompanied by pain. The techniques which are used often have an effect on groups of joints and their surrounding tissues. Regional mobilisation involves gentle and repeated passive movement of the affected area to relieve pain and increase the range of movement.

Localised mobilisation

When pain arises from a spinal disorder, the physiotherapist locates the level of the spine producing the symptoms, and may then use localised mobilisation techniques to relieve the pain and restore the normal range of movement. Localised mobilisations consist of passive, small-range, repetitive movements.

The most vigorous of the manipulative procedures is the application of a deliberate thrust to increase joint mobility, taking the movement a little further than it goes in ordinary active movements, but within the normal passive range.

Traction

This is a longitudinal stretching force applied along the axis of the tissues and is a form of regional mobilisation. It has been known for centuries that back pain can sometimes be relieved in this way. It is not known, however, why traction works when it does. Some practitioners have claimed that pulling the vertebral bodies slightly apart eases the pressure on a prolapsed disc. But this in itself would not make the extruded disc material shrink back, or repair the ruptured outer casing. One theory was that the vacuum produced in the intervertebral space would withdraw the extruded disc material away from the nerve, but bioengineering experiments have now shown this to be unlikely. Studies have suggested that the amount of traction necessary to achieve actual separation of vertebral bodies is far greater than that ever applied by way of pelvic traction in a physiotherapy department. Possibly, traction works by reducing tension or spasm in the back and hip muscles, or by easing the strain on the facet joints, but there is no conclusive evidence. Many people have found relief in this way, but if you are one of the people for whom it does not work, there is no point in persisting with it.

There are several ways of applying traction, involving, in many cases, the use of special apparatus. The magnitude of the pulling force, the position in which it is given and the time for which it is applied will all determine the effects of the traction. If the pain is worse afterwards, the treatment should be discontinued.

D-i-y traction by gravity

Patients are sometimes advised to use gravity by hanging by the hands from a firmly fixed rail, a cross–beam or the top of a door frame, if they can do so safely and conveniently at home. Gripping the top of the door, or the door frame, they gradually raise their feet off the floor by bending their knees. This exercise applies traction to the shoulder joints as well as the spine.

Movement

Exercise techniques are nearly always important in the treatment of spinal conditions. They may be used as an adjunct to mobilising procedures, to enable the patient to maintain the restored range of movement and to strengthen muscles which have become weak through disuse or inhibition by pain.

Assisted or resisted exercises

Joints can become stiff if the muscles which move them are weak; by strengthening these, mobility can be increased. Since each joint movement involves the tensing of a set of muscles and the relaxation of the opposing set, assisted and resisted movement strengthens the muscle by working it in both directions of movement. Assisted movement is when you work your muscles but the therapist helps with the range and direction; resisted movement is when the therapist pushes against you doing the movement.

Proprioceptive neuromuscular facilitation (PNF)

PNF is a system of exercise which aims to obtain maximum muscle activity by using sensory and auditory stimuli to increase the response of the neuromuscular system. Resistance and stretch are also applied to groups of muscles.

In essence, the patient performs or tries to perform movements against the manual resistance offered by the therapist in certain spiral and diagonal patterns of movement. The movements contain elements of flexion (or extension) together with a rotatory component, and are closely related to normal functional movement. Maximum contraction of strong muscles is used to reinforce the effort of weaker muscles in the pattern. The specific placing of hands to apply pressure, the use of the voice to stimulate 'push' or 'pull' and the stretching of muscles to initiate movement are stimuli used to encourage movement. PNF procedures are normally done with the patient lying supine. It is hard work for therapist and patient.

Active exercises

These are of various kinds in which the patient takes over, following the therapist's instructions, in trying to mobilise joints and strengthen muscles.

The type of exercise prescribed depends on the patient's condition, on how long he or she has been out of action and how fit he or she needs to be to return to normal life. What is suitable for one patient is not necessarily right for another.

If any exercise causes pain, it may be aggravating the condition: tell the physiotherapist when you find a movement painful. The exercise may have to be adjusted accordingly.

Some exercises are designed to strengthen and mobilise the spine when it is extended. Others strengthen the abdominal muscles; sideways bending and rotation (twisting) help to mobilise the spine. To do this, the therapist may provide manual or other resistance to particular movements. Spinal exercises are sometimes given in a hydrotherapy pool in warm water.

Some physiotherapy departments adopt the 'back school' approach in which exercises are carried out in groups. Classes with others help to raise morale, and individuals can encourage and support each other. The competition often has a stimulating effect. Physiotherapists try to ensure that exercises match the age and needs of the individual.

If you have been taught to do the exercises and are expected to do them at home, make sure that you do them. They should be done regularly and carefully, and for short periods at a time – if you have forgotten to do your morning session, do not do twice as much in the evening to catch up. Doing exercises to music or while listening to a regular radio programme may help to remind and motivate you. If rest is suggested during or after a set of exercises, this is important and should not be skimped.

Isometric exercises

It is possible to contract the muscles very strongly but not move the joints at all; this happens in arm wrestling. This muscle action is called isometric exercise and has a particular benefit for back pain. Where inflammation of joints makes moving them painful, a special range of isometric exercises can be used which strengthen the muscles by bracing them without moving joints.

Electrotherapy

Physiotherapists are trained to administer several sorts of treatment which depend on the use of different types of electrical or electronic apparatus. Many people have found these therapies beneficial in relieving pain, though the effect is in some cases short-lived.

Ultrasound
This is used in treating injury to muscles, tendons and ligaments, but not bones. Ultrasonic therapy uses the energy of sound waves at very high frequencies, inaudible to human beings. The waves are applied to the affected area through special apparatus. They penetrate the skin painlessly, help to relax muscular spasm, reduce swelling and relieve pain; they also promote healing in the tissue.

TENS (transcutaneous electrical nerve stimulation)
Severe chronic pain can sometimes be relieved by applying very small electrical currents to either side of the pain site. Like acupuncture, this method is thought to work by stimulating the nerve ends in the skin, thus overriding the nervous system's perception of pain messages.

Sufferers can administer this treatment to themselves, by means of a portable battery-operated unit, connected to electrodes which are attached to the skin with self-adhesive pads. Such units cost from £40 upwards (some physio departments and pain clinics might loan them out). The wearer can switch the current on at any time and control the amount, duration and strength of each dose of stimulation, which is felt as a gentle tingling. TENS is sometimes applied to a patient on complete bed rest. Some back pain sufferers swear by TENS, but it does not work for everybody. It is essential not to use a TENS machine unless you have seen a physiotherapist or another health professional because its use may mask pain, the cause of which should be investigated.

Interferential therapy
This is another method of using electric current, via electrodes attached to the skin around the painful area, to relieve pain by blocking the pain reception network, and to reduce inflammation by promoting better circulation. It may also be used to stimulate muscle contractions by applying a different frequency. The patient feels a tingling sensation, as in TENS.

Which kind of physiotherapy?

It is rare for a therapist to practise the full range of techniques. Some concentrate on gradual mobilisation, others on localised thrust manoeuvres, and yet others teach their patients to do active exercises. Each of these methods is beneficial to some patients, and found painful or troublesome by others.

Techniques of physiotherapeutic treatment are constantly being abandoned and resurrected and new ones appear regularly. Objective comparisons of different techniques are difficult: each one may work for some people but not for others.

Other methods

Nowadays, people are requesting the use of complementary therapies such as acupuncture and reflexology. Many fully qualified physiotherapists have developed their skills further and embraced other techniques, particularly those that have fallen into the category of alternative therapies. These include: acupuncture, aromatherapy, cranio sacral therapy and shiatsu massage.

One advantage of going to chartered physiotherapists for these types of therapy is that they are trained to degree standard and are backed by a professional code of conduct.

CHAPTER 11

COMPLEMENTARY THERAPIES

MANY people seeking relief from back pain try therapies which do not form part of orthodox medicine (although a number of conventional doctors have had training and practise them as a speciality).

You do not need to go through your GP to see an acupuncturist, osteopath, chiropractor, naturopath or shiatsu practitioner. However, if you decide to go directly to one of these therapists, it may be wise to consult your GP first, to ensure that there is no medical contra-indication in your case. However, the therapist should tell you if your condition is not suitable for the treatment in question and that you ought to be seen by a doctor.

Practitioners in private practice can charge whatever fees they choose, so you should ask beforehand what the charge is likely to be for your course of treatment.

Manipulative therapies

In some circumstances, manipulation is inadvisable or even dangerous, for example in the case of rheumatoid arthritis in the neck or an undiagnosed tumour.

Osteopathy and chiropractic are the main manipulative therapies used in treating the joints of the spine. In both, the first consultation may last an hour (and X-rays may be taken). The patient is thoroughly examined, asked to undertake a whole range of movements, and the practitioner generally asks for details of the patient's medical – and life – history. Although manipulation forms the major treatment method of both osteopaths and chiropractors, these professions also make use of other approaches such as muscle re-education and the correction of postural faults.

Osteopathy

Osteopathy is a relatively new discipline, with its roots in late-nineteenth-century America. Its founder, Andrew Taylor Still, was unhappy with the then primitive drug and surgical therapies of conventional medicine. Some of the concepts of osteopathy subsequently came across the Atlantic, and the first school in Britain was founded in London in 1917. Osteopathy complements rather than competes with conventional medicine; the GP or physician's main forms of treatment often revolve around the use of drugs, whilst osteopaths adopt the mechanical approach (concentrating on the musculo-skeletal system: the bones, joints, tendons, muscles, ligaments etc.). Using their knowledge of anatomy and physiology, osteopaths try to recognise and correct problems in body mechanics.

Treatment

Most osteopathic treatment is usually available privately, so fees will vary between practitioners and areas: find out the fees in advance before enrolling in any treatment. Many private health insurance schemes will recognise and pay for private osteopathy, so it is worthwhile checking your insurance company's rules and regulations. With the development of fund-holding in recent years, general practices are purchasing the services of osteopaths for the benefit of their patients, so the treatment is now available on the NHS. If you are referred to an osteopath within the NHS, it is likely that you will require a referral letter from your GP. In private practice you can self-refer, but check the credentials of the osteopath first and make sure that he or she is registered.

The first consultation will be similar to one with a conventional doctor: a full history will be taken and a physical examination carried out. A registered osteopath will be trained to identify any problem that is more appropriate for a doctor to deal with and will refer you if necessary. He or she will assess the posture, the state of the joints, ligaments and tendons to identify the problem. Treatment is mainly by manipulation, stretching of soft tissues, and passive movements of the back. In some cases it may be necessary to mobilise a restricted joint by thrust techniques; generally, the treatment is not uncomfortable. It has been estimated that over 5 million people consult the 2,500 practising osteopaths every year in Britain. They have treated many backache sufferers where conventional medicine has failed.

Training and regulation

There are currently five voluntary bodies which regulate the activities of osteopaths. Membership and registration of such organisations implies that they are bound by a code of conduct and are subject to disciplinary procedures. Ask which professional body your osteopath belongs to and ensure that he or she is registered.

Under the Osteopaths Act of 1993, a new General Osteopathic Council is being set up which will eventually replace the existing system and maintain a register of recognised practitioners. This should mean that osteopaths' patients will have the same assurances of professional regulation that apply to doctors and dentists.

Osteopaths can often be recognised from their qualifications: DO (Diploma of Osteopathy) or BSc (Ost) appear after their names. They have rigorous training in anatomy and physiology, bio-mechanics and relevant areas of sociology and psychology. Training focuses on the musculo-skeletal system, with emphasis on developing the practical skills for both diagnosis and treatment.

They often advertise in the *Yellow Pages* but a useful source of information is the **Osteopathic Information Service***, which has access to information about practising osteopaths in Britain and their registration status.

Chiropractic

Like osteopathy, chiropractic uses manipulative techniques to help backache sufferers; its origins also lie in late-nineteenth-century America. The word chiropractic means 'done by hand' or 'manipulation'. In global terms, it is the third largest primary health-care profession in the western world, after medicine and dentistry. However, in Britain there are only about 1,000 practitioners, under half the number of osteopaths.

Chiropractic differs from osteopathy in that chiropractors are more likely to use X-rays to determine the cause of the problem, and they often have X-ray equipment on site. They also rely less on soft-tissue and massaging techniques.

Treatment

The discipline of chiropractic is one of diagnosis followed by manipulative treatment. Chiropractors practise on the principle that poor alignment of the vertebral bodies can irritate a nerve. This resulting pressure causes symptoms such as referred pain. By manipulating the spinal column, chiropractors believe they can restore normal function; such manipulation is given to specific joints in order to relieve mechanical stress. In addition, chiropractors will give their patients individual advice about their life-style and work practices, to try to prevent the problem recurring. As in any other clinical discipline, the chiropractor will take a full history and carry out a relevant physical examination, with particular emphasis on specific joints; an X-ray will be taken if appropriate. A registered chiropractor will not treat you if the problem is inappropriate or best managed by someone else; they will refer you on to the most suitable person.

Training and registration

One recognised way to qualify as a chiropractor is to enrol in an academic course that leads to a BSc degree, followed by a post-graduate course at a recognised clinic. Only after this will the newly-qualified chiropractor be given full membership of the **British Chiropractic Association***. Check with the association that your chiropractor is appropriately qualified.

Under the Chiropractors Act of 1994 a registration council, the General Chiropractic Council, will be the sole registration body of chiropractors and will act in a similar fashion to the General Medical Council. It will control educational standards and enforce a disciplinary code of conduct.

Like osteopathy, chiropractic services are mainly available in the private sector, but some GP fund-holding practices are beginning to make such services available to their patients. You do not need your GP's permission to see a chiropractor privately, although you may wish to discuss the pros and cons of going to see a practitioner with your GP. Check in advance what the fee will be and, if you have private medical insurance, check that the services of a chiropractor are covered by the policy.

Other complementary therapies useful in the treatment of backache

Naturopathy
Naturopathy is based on the belief that healing depends on the corrective action of the body to heal itself. Naturopaths believe that illness happens as a result of toxins accumulating within the system and that the body is the best healer, so they tend to discourage drug treatment.

Acupuncture
Acupuncture is an ancient Chinese therapy used in the treatment of pain relief as well as many other diseases. The principle of acupuncture is based on the belief that in human tissue there are numerous points connected with particular organs, and that these points are linked by a network of channels, called meridians, through which streams of life-energy flow. The functioning of an organ is said to be affected by tapping these channels at appropriate points; fine needles are inserted. Other ways of tapping the points include touch (acupressure), electric currents, ultrasound and laser (see *shiatsu*).

Western medicine rests on totally different assumptions, believing that the probable explanation is that acupuncture leads the brain to produce substances called endorphins, which act as natural painkillers.

Treatment
During the initial consultation, the acupuncturist will take a detailed history of the problem. This will help to tell him or her about the condition of the body and where the life energies need to be changed. Having decided on the nature of the problem, the acupuncturist will insert the needles into sites, carefully chosen according to the type of problem the patient has. Several needles may be used at once and inserted into various depths. They can

be left in place for about half an hour, depending on the desired therapeutic effect. Sometimes they are inserted into areas far away from the site of the symptoms. The procedure is not generally uncomfortable, but if you are anxious about your first treatment you might want to take a friend with you. Most people find the treatment session relaxing and soothing.

The frequency of the treatment will vary and, like any therapeutic intervention, the response and success rate can differ enormously from person to person. There is no definite treatment span but it is not uncommon to have sessions once or twice a week. Occasionally a patient may respond dramatically, but more usually it is necessary for the treatment to span several months. Many prospective patients are concerned about the transmission of infection via acupuncture needles, but all acupuncture therapists should adhere to strict rules regarding hygiene procedures laid down by the **British Acupuncture Council★**.

Shiatsu

This is a technique that involves the application of pressure on acupuncture points and meridians. According to oriental medicine, deep pressure applied to certain points will have a similar effect to the use of needles, although the points may differ. Shiatsu was originally the Japanese form of Chinese acupuncture (see above), but has now developed techniques of its own.

Treatment will be given by exerting pressure on several specific points, as well as general kneading massage. Pressure is applied in a variety of ways: sometimes the thumb or fingers are used, sometimes the palm or heel of the hand, or a knee or elbow. The intensity of pressure varies from very gentle to very strong, but no more pain should be felt than that involved in the release of tension. By calming or exciting the selected pressure points, it has been claimed that shiatsu re-balances the body's electro-magnetic forces, which helps to enhance health and the healing processes. Contact the **Shiatsu Society★** for advice.

Aromatherapy

Aromatherapy has been with us for many centuries and involves the treatment of health problems with scented concentrated oils extracted from many different sectors of the plant and tree kingdoms. These oils are thought to have therapeutic and healing properties and can be applied via the use of massage; some can be swallowed, inhaled or used in compresses. Oils are selected individually on the basis of what you have told the therapist and from what he or she has observed and deduced from the assessment. One word of warning: do not place undiluted oils on to the skin as they can cause an allergic reaction.

Homeopathy

This is a form of therapeutics that has been around for nearly 200 years. Homeopaths use substances from plants, minerals or even animals, often in tiny doses, to boost the body's own natural defences. These medicines are chosen specifically for their ability, in much higher doses, to cause symptoms similar to those that the person already has. Although we do not fully understand how homeopathic medicines work, there is some evidence for their efficacy, and the small doses of drugs used make the procedure pretty safe. Many health practitioners, including doctors, dentists and vets, practise homeopathy.

Holistic medicine

Conventional medicine has had much criticism: one of the main ones – and with some justification – is that it fails to look at the patient as a whole person. Instead of assessing the individual and his or her environment and emotions, some doctors may concentrate solely on the disease state. The term holistic medicine has become fashionable in the last few years, promoting total health care for an individual person; this can be used with mainstream medicine, but it also embraces other disciplines such as astrology, faith healing, homeopathy and yoga. Back pain is not just a physical process and it involves emotional and mental processes which can be overlooked by conventional doctors; hence some people are attracted to complementary medicine. Some disciplines have not been scientifically validated, however, but, equally, the same criticism can be aimed at some conventional medical techniques.

Always check out any practitioner you go to. One useful starting point is the **Institute for Complementary**

Medicine*; enclose a stamped addressed envelope with two loose first-class stamps to cover costs. They are a useful umbrella source for many complementary disciplines.

CHAPTER 12

SURGERY

DOCTORS seldom suggest surgery where some other treatment remains to be tried. Spinal surgery is usually the last resort and should never be agreed to without serious consideration. To put the incidence of surgical intervention into perspective: it has been estimated that four operations will be needed for every 10,000 episodes of back pain.

No surgeon can ever guarantee prior to a spinal operation that it will be a success, and complications, some serious, can occur. The surgeon (back surgery is usually performed by an orthopaedic surgeon or a neurosurgeon, both of whom often specialise in the field of spinal surgery) should discuss the position with you fully, and should give you some idea of what to expect after the operation. No operation can be done without your consent, and a surgeon is unlikely to suggest it unless he or she is sure of your full cooperation at all stages. To a large extent, success will call for your determination to regain strength and get back to normal.

That the operation may be considered successful does not mean that the spine will be as good as new, and that all previous activities can be resumed, including ones that caused the original damage.

The spine is a complex structure and it is seldom that damage such as a disc prolapse happens in isolation. It also usually causes damage to other structures, which will not be cured by the operation and may go on causing problems afterwards. A complete recovery following a spinal operation is most likely when the damage is the result of a single incident, and not the culmination of years of gradual deterioration.

If surgery is not successful, be wary of agreeing to a second operation; statistics show that the chances of success decline with each additional one.

Who will be selected for surgery?

An operation should be used as the very last resort in back pain treatment as success cannot be guaranteed and unnecessary surgery can cause more harm than good. The decision to operate should not be made unless there is a specific, precise reason, such as: if there is severe, unremitting pain which is not responding to treatment; if there has been no improvement in the symptoms of a disc problem (usually six weeks after it began); if it has been deemed that medical treatment has failed; if there are signs of a disc prolapse; if a significant neurological defect has occurred due to pressure on the nerve, and the situation is continuing to deteriorate; if the patient is suffering from symptoms of spinal stenosis.

Emergency intervention becomes necessary if there is strong evidence that a disc or any other impingement is pressing on the cauda equina (the tail end of the spinal cord). The symptoms include loss of control of the bladder, sciatica-type pain down both legs, and numbness around the groin area.

Before any form of operation, the surgeon will want to have a firm idea of what is causing the pain. Those patients who are potential candidates for surgery will be required to undergo detailed investigations; usually more than one imaging technique will be employed to give the surgeon maximum information, for example the position of a prolapsed disc should be localised by clinical examination, then be confirmed by sophisticated imaging techniques such as a CT scan, myelography and possibly an MRI scan. Other investigations may also be ordered, depending on the problem. Simple, non-surgical measures should always be tried before surgery, and if it is not possible to diagnose the cause accurately, the necessity of the operation should be seriously questioned.

Discectomy
This operation is performed in order to free a nerve root and is done under general anaesthesia. The removal of the prolapsed

disc material may be all that is necessary, although the surgeon may decide to take out the whole of the disc, to prevent another prolapse. The surgeon makes an incision in the ligamentum flavum (see Chapter 2), creating a window into the spinal canal (fenestration). It may be necessary to remove a bit of the lamina to improve surgical access.

Discectomy is not a serious operation and can produce immediate relief from sciatic pain. The patient is usually allowed up almost at once and is encouraged to walk and bend; sometimes it is necessary to wear a corset for a few weeks. Most people are able to return to work, if it is sedentary, within a couple of months or so; but if they do heavy work, they should stay away for at least three, or possibly more, months.

In a few centres, orthopaedic surgeons and microsurgeons are speeding up recovery by doing the operation through a small cut. This technique, called microdiscectomy, can be technically more difficult to carry out but the results are encouraging. Because there is less disruption to the spine and the surrounding tissues, the recovery period is shorter, and the patient returns to his or her previous activity levels a lot more quickly.

Sometimes the surgeon finds it necessary to remove bone thickening and osteophytes from the vertebral arch or body, if they are causing stretching, angulation, adhesion or compression of the nerve roots.

Spinal fusion

This operation is designed to stiffen a section of the spine, to prevent a deformity such as spondylolisthesis from increasing; to fix a section where movement is painful, such as a degenerated disc giving an abnormal pattern of movement, with secondary changes in the facet joints; or to stabilise the spine in an area weakened during surgery.

Most commonly, the operation consists of the laying down of a bone graft to increase the stability of the spine across one, two or three vertebrae. The bone for fusion is usually taken from the hip-bone; this leaves no deformity or weakness but can be painful for weeks or months after the operation.

Spinal fusion is a much more serious operation than a discectomy. In the past, it meant lying in a plaster shell for a month, and in bed for up to three months. Nowadays, however, some surgeons allow patients up after a week or two, provided there is nothing to contra-indicate this; a corset may have to be worn. If the bones are fixed together with wires, rods or screws, the patient may be allowed up after a day or two.

The back muscles may take quite a while to recover from the operation and regain normal strength. Later, the patient will be given exercises by the physiotherapist to stabilise the spine and strengthen the muscles; in a few months he or she could be back to full activity. However, many patients take a year or more to recover completely. Much depends on the patient: the physiotherapist will show the way but it is up to the patient to do the work.

Convalescence

Prior to any back surgery (and any elective surgical operation) try to arrange for someone to keep an eye on you, and, particularly, to help you with household and everyday tasks once you have been discharged from hospital. If you live alone, with no immediate source of help, you may find that you cannot manage; this is a problem that many patients have to face. One alternative is to go into a convalescent home for a while, but there are very few of them and they may require payment. Community-based resources (for example, social services, home-help, district nurses, GPs) are also available, but may not be sufficient to help you if you live alone. Talk to the local social services department to see what assistance they can give you. Post-operative care, unless you have relatives or friends who can help, is quite difficult to come by, and this is something you should bear in mind when deciding whether or not to have surgery.

CHAPTER 13

OCCUPATIONAL THERAPY

PATIENTS may be referred to an occupational therapist after recovering from surgery as part of a rehabilitation programme, or after being inactive because of a prolonged spell of pain (where there is no surgery). Patients are referred to an occupational therapist in the same way that they are referred to a physiotherapist

Occupational therapy is a state-registered profession, supplementary to medicine. Occupational therapists who have completed their three or four years' training are entitled to put DipCOT or BScOT after their name, depending on where and when they qualified. In order to practise within the NHS, occupational therapists have to be on the state register; they can then put SROT after their name.

Occupational therapy is usually requested in the first instance by the consultant or another doctor, but the actual treatment is left to the discretion of the therapist. It may take the form of work, recreation or any activity that will be most effective in helping the patient to fully recover and return to work, or which will minimise the effects of permanent disability and help the patient to live with it.

How OT helps

Occupational therapy for patients with back problems is mainly re-educative: the therapist will help the patient to learn to manage his or her own body, realise the limitations imposed by the condition and avoid conditions that bring on the back pain. In addition, the patient will be taught new ways of carrying out everyday activities so as not to aggravate the condition, including how to bend and lift. Advice is also given on more suitable seating and better work positions.

In nearly all occupational therapy departments, there is an area with a kitchen, bathroom and bedroom, where patients are taught safer ways to carry out activities and then practise them under supervision until the techniques become automatic; it is not easy to change movement-patterns of a lifetime without professional help.

If the patient's house is badly designed for a person with back trouble, the occupational therapist from the hospital or from the local authority social services department may visit and recommend adaptations. The social services department may be able to provide some financial help.

The occupational therapy assessment

The occupational therapist must first become familiar with the patient's medical history: it is likely that he or she will have read through the medical records before the appointment. An understanding of body mechanics and back care, coupled with their practical experience, puts an occupational therapist in an ideal position to advise on how to cope with the problems of normal, everyday living.

The therapist will be interested in: how the patient is coping following an episode of backache or surgery; in his or her home situation, i.e. the type of house the patient has, for example, a home with stairs may present more problems than a bungalow; the patient's employment and what tasks the job may involve.

It is quite likely that the occupational therapist will work with the physiotherapist; there is a fair amount of overlap in these two fields, but generally the occupational therapist will look at the patient's functional capabilities and how they can be improved, while the physiotherapist will try to improve the patient's mobility through exercise regimes. If the backache sufferer is an in-patient, it is possible that both therapists will do a home-visit with him or her, prior to discharge from hospital, to see the home circumstances and decide how they can be improved. The occupational therapist may also work with other health professionals, such as the patient's GP, social workers and other doctors involved in the case.

The occupational therapist will appraise how the patient is coping with, for example, going to the toilet, dressing, getting in and out of the bath, bed and chairs with, or without, assistance. Once the assessment is complete, the therapist will decide what the best course of action is and will give a verbal or written report to the doctor in charge of the case.

The patient will also be given advice about correct posture, how to lift objects without excessively straining his or her back and general back care. For those people with persistent, recurrent episodes, the therapist may supply aids which will assist in daily activities, for example, a raised toilet seat, or even handrails around the toilet area, may make life much easier for more disabled people. Much of the equipment is inexpensive and simply designed; the use of long-handled shoe horns or a non-slip bath mat could, for instance, make a big difference.

Rehabilitation and returning to work

If you are still attending the hospital when you are almost fit for work, the occupational therapist may help by analysing your job requirements and suggesting ways of lessening back strain.

Some employers are quite progressive and will allow you to return to work when you are nearly completely better, offering you lighter duties to start with, then slowly returning you to your previous role. Often you will be required to see the company doctor (if there is one) to ascertain your fitness for work, or if you are considering leaving work on the grounds of ill health. If there is no company doctor, it is likely that the personnel officer or immediate superior will take an interest. The employers may also want medical information about your illness in order to assess your fitness for work. They may consider contacting your GP or specialist, usually requesting a written medical report. Under the Access to Medical Records Act, you will be informed of this action and you must give written consent to your employers before they approach the doctor. The doctor will not communicate with the company unless he or she has your written consent. Your employers should also inform you of your rights, under the act, which include the right to see the medical report, before it is sent off to them. Any costs of obtaining such a medical report are usually met by them.

If your doctor considers you unfit for any form of employment, he or she will issue you with a DSS sick note, for which there is no fee. However, the doctor may charge you for filling in any insurance claim forms that you may have in connection with your illness. Some people will qualify for welfare benefits if they are particularly disabled. It might be worth talking to your local Citizens Advice Bureau if you are having problems or need help with welfare benefits.

CHAPTER 14

PREVENTING A RECURRENCE

FOR people who have already experienced one episode of back trouble, the probability of being struck by an acute attack of back pain is higher than for people who have never yet been troubled. This is because an attack, regardless of what caused it, tends to leave the victim with a degree of tissue damage, or with weaker back and abdominal muscles than before.

Back schools

There are a growing number of back schools, usually attached to physiotherapy departments in hospitals. They offer a form of educational therapy first developed in Sweden for back-pain sufferers. It consists of instruction on how to use the body actively and posturally, the anatomy of the spine, and descriptions of the causes of back pain. Advice on the layout, planning and design of work – ergonomics – is also given. The lesson is simple: the better you understand your back, the more readily you can cope when it is painful. The proponents of such back schools feel that their approach is just as good as many other treatments; certainly there is no obvious harm in using these techniques.

Advice on posture

Many of us acquire minor postural deformities which lead to avoidable backache (which can be treated), for example the tendency to a rounded back, head poked forward and shoulders tensed up. If this is due to muscular weakness and stiffness, exercises should help. But often it is just a matter of habit; old

101

habits should therefore be shed and new ones learned, and postural advice on a new way of using your body can help.

The Alexander Technique

The Alexander Technique is a method of postural re-education. Fundamental to the technique, which is over 100 years old, is the concept of 'use' of the body. Rather than focusing on specific problems (e.g. back pain), the overall use of the body is looked at, and the aim is to increase the pupil's awareness of balance, poise and movement in everyday activity. For example, habitual slouching when sitting would be seen as harmful body use. It is believed that for each of us there is an optimum posture and way of moving. This unfortunately becomes overlaid with bad habits which then feel natural to us. The task of the Alexander teacher is to make the pupil more aware of his or her physical self, to enable him or her to direct the mind or body towards using it in a better way.

In practice, the Alexander Technique is taught by a teacher encouraging small physical adjustments to the pupil's body but not in the way that a manipulator such as a chiropractor would. The teacher uses his or her hands to try to promote a specific type of muscle tone, coupled with verbal instructions. These lessons enable the pupil to gain experience of an easier and freer way of movement.

The Alexander Technique is taught on a one-to-one basis, as people have individual habits, but it is possible to find group classes which give a general idea of how the technique works; some adult education institutes run such courses. The cost of the courses vary, depending on the area of the country, but they are roughly comparable with the price of an equivalent session with an osteopath or chiropractor or other alternative therapists. Occasionally some teachers will talk to the patient, free of charge, as a means of introduction. There are 600 specialist teachers in Britain; they have to have a full-time, three-year training course and reach a standard that permits them to become teaching members of the **Society of Teachers of the Alexander Technique★** (STAT).

Feldenkrais Method

The Feldenkrais Method is concerned with creating a greater awareness of patterns of movement, the aim being a gradual re-education leading to greater freedom of movement and enhanced comfort. The method has its roots in Western science (physics and mechanical engineering) and Eastern martial arts (judo), as its founder, Dr Moshe Feldenkrais, was highly trained in both. The focus is on learning to recognise ways of moving or holding the body which are restrictive and habitual, and on discovering new options which are more efficient and graceful. The re-learning process is facilitated by the use of gentle movements, done at a pace and intensity that does not involve force or pain. The lessons usually begin lying or sitting on the floor and involve new perceptions of walking, crawling, the natural movements of babies, awareness of breathing while moving and the way in which the head, eyes, spine and limbs move in relation to one another.

The method is taught in two different formats: as a series of lessons, called Awareness through Movement, through which a teacher leads a group in classes and workshops; and as one-to-one lessons called Functional Integration. People who learn this method are described as students rather than patients, reinforcing the principle that this is an educational process. Another way of trying to understand the method is to compare the Feldenkrais Method, with, for example, chiropractic. The latter is done by altering structure (the musculo-skeletal) through manipulation. The Feldenkrais method works with your ability to alter and regulate your movement. In this case the brain is targeted, not the skeleton and its associated structures. To obtain a directory of teachers (there are about 35 accredited members of the Feldenkrais Guild) and further information contact the **Feldenkrais Guild★**.

Signs and warnings
Having once been afflicted with back pain, you should be able to recognise some of the danger signs: perhaps a stab of pain in a muscle, or a tingling in the fingers or toes, warning you that you must stop what you are doing, or change some posture you are maintaining. If you know of something in your daily routine that triggered off the original trouble, and you have not changed your ways, do so now. This may involve changing your leisure activities, or your job, temporarily, or even permanently. Even if

this possibility raises great difficulties, it needs to be considered seriously. Traditionally, it is thought that people who refuse to 'give in' to back pain are the very ones who are most likely to be plagued by repeated attacks. This could result in the underlying condition, which caused the attacks, becoming chronic. (In medical language, chronic means long-term, see Chapter 17.)

Another approach used by some doctors to patients' attitude to pain is to advise tackling it more directly. Many people live in fear of pain. This is perfectly normal and understandable but, as pain is a common experience, exaggerated fears may need investigation and unravelling. The medical profession itself has tended to encourage people's fear of pain, advising rest when, perhaps, encouragement to become active again might have been wiser.

The chronic sufferer

When certain changes have occurred in the structure of the spine, especially if they are the outcome of a degenerative process, there is no way of restoring all the functions or a normal spine.

Sometimes people have to be told that there is nothing more that can be done in the way of medical treatment for their back trouble, and find that treatment by physiotherapists or other therapists does not ease their suffering; they must then learn to live with their faulty spine.

Such advice is bound to be depressing. Moreover, chronic pain itself can be depressing. Some people in this situation let the rest of their life be dominated by their back trouble; others are more able to meet the challenge and learn to cope.

Try anything

Although a patient may have been told that all the normal measures have been tried, there is always a possibility that the verdict may become outdated by new knowledge, improved diagnostic techniques and methods of treatment not previously available.

Some sufferers, therefore, feel that there is always a chance that another surgeon, another doctor, another therapist, may have a way of doing something for them. There are a number of doctors and other therapists in private practice who offer specialist treatment for back pain. Sometimes they are exponents of a particular line of therapy, and if that does not work are therefore unlikely to propose alternatives. The main advantage in seeing someone privately is that the patient may be seen more quickly and may be buying more time with the particular practitioner. Time seems to be an important factor in determining patient satisfaction with a therapist, regardless of what the therapy is. Many backache sufferers complain that they have not been given enough time to deal with their problem and as a result can be dissatisfied with the treatment, irrespective of how well it should work on paper. Doctors in private medical practice and complementary therapists tend to spend more time with the patient.

Making the best of things

A chronic back-pain sufferer can do much to help him or herself. First of all, there are almost certainly alternative ways of tackling any particular job which cause less spinal stress and are therefore less painful, and which are physically more efficient. Also, it is possible to alter or redesign your working environment with the aim of minimising postural stress on the spine: by adjusting the height of a working surface, by changing your own posture, by choosing a different chair or desk.

There are a number of aids to back comfort, some designed for the disabled, which can be used to make life more independent. **The Disabled Living Foundation★** can provide information on what special equipment is available and where it can be obtained.

The **National Back Pain Association★** is a registered charity whose aim is to promote research into the causes, treatments and prevention of back pain, and to increase understanding of how the problem of back pain can be avoided. The membership fee of £15 (and concession of £7.50 for pensioners and those on welfare benefits) a year includes subscription to a quarterly magazine, *Talkback*, with information about the association's activities and research projects, and other relevant publications. Local groups of back pain sufferers have been set up in some places under the NBPA's auspices.

Pain clinics
If you have chronic back pain which you are finding hard to cope with, your GP or specialist may refer you to a pain clinic run under the auspices of the NHS. A number of services are offered at such a clinic, although the particular range varies from area to area. Advice on painkilling drugs will be given, and suitable physiotherapy techniques, occupational therapy, and counselling may also be available as well as highly specialised techniques of pain relief such as epidural injections. Many pain clinics will loan out equipment such as TENS machines. These clinics are often run by anaesthetists who have a special interest in pain relief regardless of the cause. Contact **Pain Concern UK*** for advice.

What you can do to help yourself
It is important to identify the things that do not make matters worse, and concentrate on them as a basis for an improvement of life. Assuming you can find some activity – such as short walks or swimming, or simple exercises which do not upset your back – do it regularly, a bit more and a bit faster or further every day. Almost any exercise (not jogging) will do to start with, as the basis for improvement and to help you to become generally fitter.

People who are physically fit can usually tolerate pain better than unfit people. The sensation of pain may be no different but it affects them less and they are better able to ignore it.

Some of the things you can do which should make your life easier include:

- keep a check on your weight; extra pounds mean extra stress on the spine
- eat a healthy, balanced diet
- learn to relax (use music or audio tape with a progressive muscular régime)
- learn to live according to a routine and plan ahead, so that you never need to rush
- give careful consideration to the movements or actions that aggravate your symptoms, and try to avoid them

- when you have a 'good' day, do not try to catch up on all the neglected things: having further weeks of misery because you rushed to do too much on the 'good' day is not worth it
- make sure that you have a suitable chair and bed – ask advice from the physiotherapist, occupational therapist, osteopath or chiropractor before buying new furniture
- keep active. Rest is appropriate for acute back pain for a short time-span, such as 48 hours; chronic back pain tends to benefit from the right kind of exercise, preferably of the most enjoyable type and as strenuous as you can manage
- change patterns and positions as needed to ensure that your sex life can continue on as regular a basis as possible. Prolonged back pain can have a devastating effect on sexual activity. Back pain can also be used (often unconsciously) as an excuse for not engaging in sexual activity. The situation deserves understanding and sympathetic analysis from both partners, with no pressure to perform. Postures can be experimented with, for example, which partner is on top; side to side positions; one partner sitting on a chair, the other astride.

The future for back trouble

Back trouble – chiefly in the form of low back pain – has taken on some aspects of an epidemic in the Western world; that is to say, though it is not an infectious complaint, its incidence is seen to be constantly increasing. In Britain, it creates a demand for treatment which represents an ever-increasing burden on the health services. If this rate of growth of backache continues, it will have a dramatic effect on the funding of health care. Over the last few years, many countries have looked at their ever-expanding health bill and have tried to trim health budgets. In such a tough economic climate, backache, which has always had a poor public-relations image, is likely to suffer. Such a squeeze of funding may have profound implications in the way that backache is managed.

It would seem, therefore, that back-pain sufferers of the future are more likely to be offered short shrift and grudging sympathy by doctors and employers alike. Harsh though this may seem, it has some backing from some advanced medical opinion.

Pain avoidance and pain confrontation

The latest approaches to the problem of back pain take their stand on the fact that most back pain is self-limiting; in 80 to 90 per cent of cases, an attack will clear up within six weeks at the most, whether it is left alone or treated, and regardless of the form that any treatment takes.

Nor, it is claimed, does it make much difference whether the patient adopts the method of inactivity (referred to as 'pain avoidance') or simply carries on with his or her usual activities as best he or she can (called 'pain confrontation'). Recovery is said to be, if anything, more likely to be rapid with the latter approach.

The disability factor

Back pain, from this point of view, is not really on the increase. What is increasing to epidemic proportions is people's readiness to expect medical treatment for it and increased incidence of 'back pain disability' – an illness in which psychological factors play as important a part as physical ones. It manifests itself in acceptance of invalidity, which means staying away from work, retiring to bed, requesting sickness certificates and extensive treatment. It is a self-reinforcing condition in that the more the sufferer gives way to it and comes to see him or herself as an invalid, the worse the chances of recovery.

This is even more the case if the patient undergoes a variety of treatments, including surgery, which fail to bring about satisfactory relief; each successive treatment carries a reduced chance of success and leads to a further retreat into invalidism.

It is pointed out that with improvements in medical care in less advanced parts of the world, back pain disability increases because people who would previously have had to put up with their discomfort until it went away are now encouraged to seek medical help in the hope of immediate relief or cure.

Attitudes to pain

At the root of this search for medical help is said to be the psychological problem of the fear of pain. Attitudes to pain are highly subjective, and conditioned by the individual's psychology, which is the product of many different factors. Thus, tolerance of pain varies enormously, and an identical kind of pain provokes widely different reactions.

The confrontationalists believe that an acute condition is most likely to become chronic in people who are least able or willing to tolerate pain, because prolonged rest and the avoidance of exertion are not curative, but debilitating. Muscles, joints and bones deteriorate so that each activity becomes progressively harder, forming a vicious circle; and a weakened physique also predisposes to further injury. Psychologically, too, the motivation towards effort becomes progressively fainter.

So the treatment of back pain in the future seems likely to take the form of encouraging the patient to refuse to give way to his or her pain, and, by so doing, to limit its duration and effect.

It is obvious that there is a close interplay between attitudes towards pain, symptoms of backache and the degree of disability. Sometimes people with chronic backache develop a depressive illness which may exacerbate the reaction towards pain. If the patient is feeling anxious, for whatever reason, the symptoms may well be made worse. Often, psychological intervention in the form of seeing a therapist, with or without drug treatment, may help the psychological problems and hence the response to pain.

Another problem not uncommonly seen is the adoption of the sick role in someone who has had extensive medical tests and treatments. This group of people have often seen many doctors and, perhaps, complementary therapists. Sometimes it may be necessary to cease all active intervention and just remain on the minimum of essential therapy. The mind is very powerful, and the role it plays in backache sufferers' rehabilitation, although not fully understood, is extremely important.

CHAPTER 15

TAKING CARE OF YOUR BACK

FEW people give a thought to their spine until they are suffering the consequences of not thinking. When you find yourself squatting to reach a low cupboard because you cannot bend your aching back, you become aware that you should have learned to squat in the first place.

Everyone should learn the basic rules of looking after the spine. If you have never felt so much as a twinge, following these rules should help to ensure that you never will. If you have already suffered a bout of back trouble, they should help to prevent recurrences.

If this trouble has left you with some permanent problem, you will hardly need telling to treat your back with respect. But if you now feel perfectly all right, 'as good as new', avoid the false optimism of thinking you can now resume all your old ways. Once you have had back trouble, you are rather more likely to have it again unless you take deliberate measures to prevent it.

This is not to say that you should become excessively anxious about yourself, or avoid every sort of activity. On the contrary, it is important that you should be as active as possible.

Without physical activity, the body becomes weak and unstable, and without movement it becomes stiff. The mobility of the spine and the resilience of its joints and ligaments are essential functions. Without them, the spine would be more readily strained and would lose its shock-absorbing capacity. Even more important are the muscles; not only those of the back but all those which support the spine, including the abdominal muscles. Without muscular support, the spine is unstable and easily injured.

Every one of your daily activities needs to be reviewed in the light of what you know about the structures of your back, and how they are affected by bending, twisting, and even keeping still.

Lying in bed

If you never need to give your back a thought when you wake up in the morning; if there is no stiffness or pain when you roll over, sit up, and get out of bed, then your bed is probably all right for you – no matter how it looks to other people.

But if you wake up with a feeling of stiffness which does not disperse until you have been moving around for a while, the cause may simply be your bed.

Mattress

A very soft or sagging mattress makes your vertebral column sag, stretching the ligaments that support it. This matters less if you change position frequently in your sleep, but if you tend to lie all night in one position, these ligaments may be strained. A soft mattress which allows you to sink deeply into it may even discourage you from moving about.

Even people whose back does not normally trouble them find that a soft bed leaves them feeling stiff in the morning. A good bed should support the body evenly, and be easy to move about on.

If you decide to buy a new bed, choose one with a firm or solid base; avoid one that is soft or springy. Choose a reasonably firm mattress: it is better to buy one which feels a little too hard, rather than one which is too soft. So-called 'orthopaedic' mattresses tend to be more expensive than ordinary firm mattresses, without having any special advantages.

If the bed you have is too soft, you can make it firmer by putting a board under the mattress, provided that the mattress itself is not disintegrating with age. The board should be as wide as the bed base and at least as long as the distance from your head to your buttocks.

Pillows

Arrange the pillows in a way that seems to you to be the most comfortable. A pillow placed between the head and shoulders needs to support the neck rather than the head. There is seldom any need to buy special pillows.

But too many pillows, or too thick a pillow, would push the head up, stretching the neck; and while you are asleep, the neck is then apt to bend sideways or forwards and the spine to become flexed. The neck vertebrae should always be kept in a continued line with the vertebrae of the chest.

Lying on your back with the head resting on a 'butterfly' pillow supports the head and stops it lolling from side to side. Simply tying a folded towel round your neck may also do the trick. (You can make a butterfly pillow by taking a thin or loosely-filled pillow and shaking the filling down each end, then twisting the pillow in the centre or tying it in half.) You may find it necessary to place another pillow underneath.

For someone who needs lots of pillows at night because of a bad chest, it is best to organise the support so that the whole spine rests on an incline. You may be able to do it with pillows; or it may be possible to incline the whole bed by raising the legs at the head on to blocks. The aim is to keep the whole spine, trunk and head in line with each other.

Getting dressed

If you are already suffering from back trouble you may find it best to wear clothes which can be put on and taken off without much bending or arm raising. Gadgets are available to help spinal sufferers with putting on difficult garments such as tights, socks and shoes. When bending down to tie shoelaces causes a problem, this can be solved by sitting on a chair with a supportive back, and bending the hip and knee to bring the foot up to within reach – that is, using hip and knee movement instead of back movement.

Standing

For a correct stance, lift the top of your head, keeping your chin tucked in. As well as standing tall, you should stand relaxed. Standing still for a long period can be uncomfortable if you are not used to it, and it is then easy to sag, so increasing the fatiguing effect by straining the muscles. However, except for soldiers on parade, standing still is rarely necessary. Mostly, we are free to look about, move our hands and shift from one foot to another, and so any given stance is seldom maintained for long. Consciously pulling in your abdomen is helpful.

One remedy for postural stress is to change position. If you cannot, and the job calls for work with one hand only, use the other hand to lean on. When you use both hands and are standing at a work bench, table or sink, ideally you should be able to rest your pelvis or stomach against it, with one foot forward in line with your hands, so that you have a balanced posture.

Washing hair and shaving

Leaning forward over a dressing-table or washbasin to see in a mirror may become a cause of backache. It can be avoided by bringing the mirror nearer, either putting it on an extension arm or fixing it on the wall beside the basin. While shaving, the fact that your arms are raised increases the workload on the back if you have to bend forward. For arranging your hair, the mirror need not be so close, but must be at a suitable height. If you have to stoop to see in the mirror, raise it further up the wall.

Bending over a basin to wash your hair puts undue stress on both the neck and the back. It may help to sit on a stool and rest your elbows on the side of the basin or sink. A better way is to wash your hair under the shower. If necessary, you can buy an inexpensive shower attachment to fit on to the bath taps, and wash your hair while bathing.

Just sitting

When sitting at leisure, the important thing is to get the buttocks well back into the chair because sitting slouched in a chair may flex the lumbar region more than any other movement or posture. Some back sufferers are more comfortable if they avoid crossing their knees and sit with their feet and knees well apart.

If the chair is soft and does not give enough support, put a cushion at the small of the back. Some people with back trouble prefer high-backed chairs, but lumbar support is more important than support at shoulder level.

Choose a chair that is the right height for you: your feet should be planted on the floor, not dangling in space. Avoid a very low chair as this can put undue strain on your back when you get up out of it.

Back shops

There are specialist shops throughout the country which supply goods (e.g. furniture, pillows) specifically for people with back problems. When possible, try something out in the shop before buying it; otherwise, see if you can buy it on approval, so you can return it if you find it is not suitable for you. The **National Back Pain Association*** produces an information sheet which lists back shops throughout Britain.

Sitting when working

The seat of the chair for working should be deep enough (front to back) so that the thighs are supported, and the front edge of the seat should not dig into the thigh; this could cause pressure on the sciatic nerve.

The back rest of a typist-chair should be adjustable so that the height above the seat can be varied to provide support at the lumbar part of the spine. Where there is a full-length back rest, it should be contoured to give support at the lumbar level.

Office work often requires both writing and typing, and each requires a different posture. Since the height of office desks can seldom be varied, it should be possible to raise and lower the chair.

Typing imposes a fair amount of strain on the back, particularly the neck and upper back, and also on the shoulders, because the typist often has to sit for longish periods with the arms unsupported. Therefore, for typing you should sit higher than for writing; the keyboard should be at a height that allows the upper arms to hang relaxed, with only the weight of the forearms having to be lifted. You should sit as close to the typewriter as you can without cramping your movements. If you sit too far from it, you have to lift the whole arm forward to reach it, increasing the strain on the upper back.

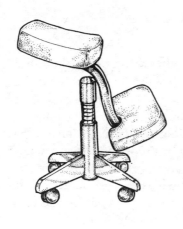 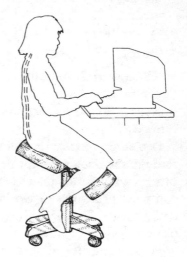

A special chair is widely available, which looks rather like a prie-dieu, but the upper cushion is for sitting on; it is tilted forward, and your knees rest on the lower cushion. There is no back support, but because some of your weight is taken by your knees and thighs, your back naturally assumes the correct lumbar curve. Chairs of this sort may be found specially comfortable when no back support is required; for example, for typing, but not all day long. Several versions are available, some with adjustable height.

Desks and other equipment

Chairs used for work are satisfactory only if the working environment in which they are used is also well designed. Even if your working chair allows you to sit supported in the right places, with the spine in a balanced neutral position and freedom to make regular minor changes in posture, the work itself may make it less than satisfactory, if ergonomics have not been taken into account.

115

For a given situation, at work or at leisure, the key factors are

- the angle of vision, and the need for subsidiary movements of the head
- the position of the hands relative to the seat and feet and
- the support of the body.

When work is laid out on a flat surface, the angle of vision is downwards, and it is necessary to bend the head. To avoid this, designers, architects, artists and draughtsmen work on tilted surfaces.

For other people, to avoid bending the head forward when reading, the book or paper needs to be propped up. Rather than sitting with head bent when paperwork such as ledgers, computer print-outs or working drawings have to be flat on the desk, it is better to lean forward supporting oneself on the table or desk with the elbows.

For writing, the desk should be high enough to allow the knees to tuck right under it, and let you sit fairly upright. But not so high as to strain the arms and shoulders; that is, not much above elbow height when sitting relaxed.

If a lot of reading or writing has to be done, a tilted desk is best. Where such a desk is not available, a drawing board propped up slantwise on books can provide a substitute. It is also possible to buy a special sloped writing surface.

Typists and VDU operators risk postural stress by repeatedly bending the neck down and sideways to look at whatever they are copying. This can be avoided if the material to be copied is raised and placed centrally – for instance, on an inclined clipboard, reading stand or lectern, behind the keyboard.

Try not to sit still for long periods; get up and walk about now and again.

Housework

With any task, in and out of the house, it is the length of time spent in any one position, as well as the effort imposed on the back, that counts. It is a good idea to change tasks (and therefore positions) fairly often. Any activity where repetitive bending is required may cause trouble, particularly if it becomes tiring.

Instead of doing one job until the bitter end, it may be possible to alternate it with another. For example, instead of spending a whole afternoon standing up ironing, leave half of it until later on, and do something else meanwhile.

If you have had back trouble, learn to delegate some or all of the heavier jobs that were formerly your lot. Make all able-bodied members of the family pull their weight.

Bed making is a job that often makes a painful back worse, and in some cases even induces back trouble, because it requires a good deal of bending and stretching. Ideally, the bed should be high enough for the mattress to be at hip height, narrow enough for you to reach across easily, and placed so that you can walk all round.

On the old-fashioned high bedstead, it requires less effort to make the bed than on a low divan bed. A low bed can be raised by putting blocks or bricks under the legs.

When making the bed, get close to it and bend at the hips and knees, keeping your back upright. If you have any difficulty in bending at hips and knees, kneel down when tucking in the bedclothes.

A fitted bottom sheet and a duvet do away with the need to bend to tuck in bedclothes. When changing a fitted sheet, do not stretch over the bed, but kneel close to each corner of the bed in turn.

A mattress should be turned by someone else. If you really have to do it yourself, have handled fitted to the sides (at the ends, too, if it is to be turned fore and aft). Grasp the handles and lift the side of the mattress so that you stand erect; back away a step and then step up on to the base and raise the mattress high enough to turn it over by letting it fall over to the other side. But it is better to leave it to other members of the household to do the turning.

Cleaning the bath puts considerable strain on the back. This job can be done much more easily by kneeling beside the bath and leaning across to rest one hand on the far edge of the bath to take your body weight, or by sitting on a chair alongside. A long-handled sponge or mop is useful. A bath is cleaned more easily when still warm immediately after use, so keep cleaning materials at hand, and insist that the others in the household clean the bath themselves.

You can avoid cleaning the bath altogether; putting a squirt of washing-up liquid in the bath water will ensure that there will be no ring.

Cleaning the floor and using a vacuum cleaner can be stressful to the back, and so do it in short sessions. Make sure that the handle is long enough for you. Some cylinder cleaners have extension pieces; fitting one of these may help. When vacuuming, use your legs and your body weight to do the work. Always pull forwards and backwards in short lengths. Avoid twisting movements. Above all, do not just stand and make your arms do the work: that way is bound to stress your back. Upright vacuum cleaners are often advised. Similarly, when using a mop, carpet sweeper or broom, move the whole body forwards and backwards with the sweeping action, instead of bending from the waist to get the increased reach.

Dusting gives you opportunities for different kinds of muscle action. It is a good idea to slot short periods of it into spells of vacuuming, polishing, washing floors or any other task which requires vigorous movement in one direction only, for which you generally use your stronger arm. Try using the other arm or use both arms and stretch upwards to counteract the bending and pushing movements of vacuuming.

In the kitchen, have at hand all the things you use regularly – for instance, saucepans on the wall, plates and dishes at waist height. Only the things you use least often, or which are fairly light, should be stowed away below thigh height in low cupboards or out of easy reach above chest height. Ideally, heavy equipment such as a food mixer or cast iron casserole should be kept where it need not be lifted to be got out.

Whenever you have to do anything near floor level, get right down to it. Bend your knees to lift dishes in and out of the oven or dishwasher. When lifting a heavy casserole, hold it close to your body, with your elbows bent. To save your back, do it in stages: put a stool at the side of the oven, squat down, put the casserole on the stool, stand up and lift the casserole on to the top of the cooker or working surface.

Having a tall stool in the kitchen is a good idea so that you can alternate between sitting and standing. A stool should have a foot-rail and needs to be of a height to suit the height of the work surface.

Work surfaces

The height of work surfaces – sink, draining board, table or working area – matters a great deal. The correct height varies with the job being done, as well as from person to person. The surface should be high enough so that you do not have to bend forwards, but not so high that you have to hunch your shoulders in order to do the job. A cooker or a kitchen unit can be raised by being put on a plinth.

If you are too tall for washing up, without stooping over the sink, raise the washing-up bowl by putting it on a small wooden stand, or on top of another upturned bowl, or on the draining board. If the surface is too high for you, try standing on a small step (made out of an inverted box, perhaps) while working there, but you could hurt yourself by forgetting about the box and stepping off unwittingly.

Ideally, it would be better to rearrange your kitchen so that the worktops are the correct height. The top of a sink should be at about elbow height, but work surfaces and the top of a cooker should be two or three inches lower. It is important to stand close to the work surface.

Less standing

You may be able to cut down on cooking: by the use of a microwave oven and a freezer, you can abolish lengthy standing at a conventional hob, do away with heavy metal saucepans, reduce washing up. Having a reserve of frozen dishes means that you can have a hot meal even when your back is playing up: but be sure to have an upright freezer, not the cavernous chest type.

Many domestic activities (preparing food, washing up, ironing) can be done seated. There is no law that says you have to stand to iron. Alter the height of the board to relate to your sitting position. It is important not to have it too high because having the arms continually raised imposes strain on the shoulders, neck and upper back.

Washing clothes

When washing by hand, do not use a sink or basin that makes you stoop: it is better to put a bowl at the right height for you in the sink or on the draining board.

Wet clothes and bed linen are much heavier than dry ones: lifting wet sheets and towels in and out of a low washing machine is the sort of movement that might eventually cause back trouble. When taking clothes out of a front-loading washing machine, put a low chair or stool beside the machine. Put a basket or large bowl on the floor and, squatting down, pull the washing into it. Then carefully lift the basket on to the stool. Do this in stages; try to make sure that you lift only one piece of wet washing at a time.

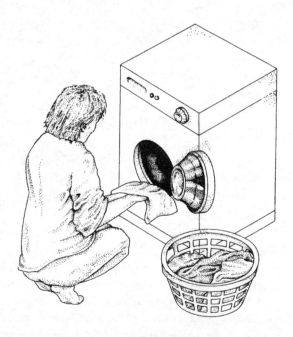

Squat with a straight back to reach low items;
e.g. to load or unload a washing machine

Looking after babies and young children

A cot with a drop-side makes it easier to lift a child in and out; choose a cot high enough to save you having to stoop. Bringing the child's weight as close to your body as possible reduces the amount of effort required.

When lifting a toddler from the ground, bend your knees to go down and lift him or her close to you. Swinging a child up at arms' length can cause acute back trouble.

With a rucksack type of baby carrier, where the child is placed behind the parent, its weight is taken through the shoulders and across the back of the hips. If possible, get someone to lift the carrier on for you, or find a safe place to prop it and the baby, while you get it on to your shoulders.

When bathing a small baby in a baby bath, put the bath on a table where you can stand or sit without stooping. Do not try to empty the bath yourself if you have a vulnerable back, because water is heavy to carry, and baby baths are an awkward shape to lift. Get an able-bodied person to do it for you. If none is available, bale out the water gradually with a jug. This will mean several trips and is laborious, but it is better than injuring your back.

When dressing a child, put him or her on a chair or bed to avoid undue bending. For doing up shoelaces, the foot should be put up on to a box or chair. Do not stoop – squat or kneel instead.

Lifting, shifting and carrying

Injuries can be caused by the unexpected: the box that was full when you thought it was empty, mistiming when lifting something jointly with another person, the load that you did not know was stuck.

The secret of safe lifting is to avoid static heaving and to use your body weight.

Stand properly: when you lift or shift an object, get as close to it as possible, with feet around it rather than to one side or behind it. Stand so that you are firmly balanced, one foot ahead of the other, ready to move off in the right direction.

To get a good grip on the load, bend the hips and knees until it can be reached, then grasp it firmly. If there is nothing on the load by which to hold it, use a sling, or ropes.

Technique of lifting

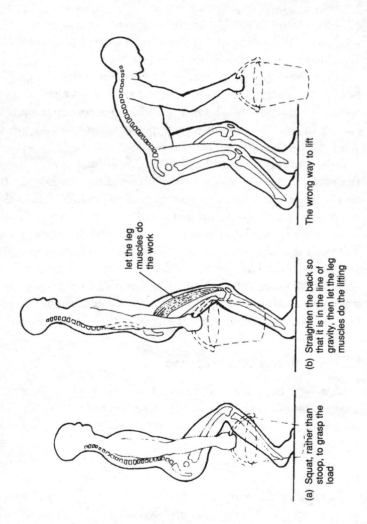

let the leg muscles do the work

(a) Squat, rather than stoop, to grasp the load

(b) Straighten the back so that it is in the line of gravity, then let the leg muscles do the lifting

The wrong way to lift

Lifting, heaving or carrying with arms outstretched throws needless strain on your chest, upper back and shoulders – so keep the load close to your body. A weight held out at arms' length causes as much stress on the spine as ten times that weight held close to the side, hence the risk when lifting a box out of a car boot. The shorter the lever, the smaller the effort required, so the closer you can get to the object, the better.

When dealing with something large and heavy, lift it first at one end only, and get it on to a higher level before you take the full load. This halves the stress.

When putting things down, if you cannot safely drop the object (which is the best way), put the lifting drill into reverse. Keep the object close to your body, watch your fingers and put one end or corner down first.

Rather than carrying a heavy load, pull it on a trolley or, if that is not possible, divide it into two smaller loads – one for each hand – or make a second journey.

Whatever you are lifting or carrying, keep its centre of gravity as near as you can over or under your own centre of gravity. This means that you have to keep your knees apart enough to keep the load close to you, and must use your leg muscles to help lift. Basically, before you actually lift, it is a good idea to check quickly that your back is in the correct posture, then look up and tuck your chin in. (Do not tackle a lifting job with your back rotated, twisted or bent sideways.)

Using your body weight can help to move things and saves the stress of direct muscular effort. If you move your body to give it momentum, it has what is called kinetic energy, and you can transfer that energy to something else. Just as you can give a cricket ball enough movement and thus kinetic energy to break a window, you can use your body in such a way that energy is transferred to the load you wish to shift. In this way, stress on the spine is reduced.

Do not ever attempt to shift a heavy cupboard or chest by yourself. If furniture has to be moved, try to get help. Unload every single item from the cupboard on to a convenient table before moving the cupboard; this is laborious but safer.

When pushing or pulling, make use of your legs and body weight. If the object to be moved is high and stable enough, you may be able to move it by leaning your back against it and pushing with your legs (wear shoes that grip the floor). If low and stable, it may be possible to move the object by lying on your back on the floor and pushing with your feet.

Ideally, all heavy pieces of furniture should have castors fitted on them to make them easy to move.

Gardening

The same rules apply to gardening jobs as to household ones: lift and carry carefully, using your legs and body weight; work upright whenever practical; do not do too much at once, and change tasks often; keep the work as close to yourself as possible; get help when necessary.

Avoid prolonged bending and stooping by kneeling down or using a long-handled implement to do the job whenever possible.

For pruning and fruit picking, long-handled implements which allow you to avoid reaching high up above, should be used with care. While they may not be heavy items in themselves, when they are lifted or lowered they put a stress on the back.

Try to keep the sweeps of action in a forward or backward direction, with the minimum of twisting. Avoid any sweeping action across the body: it needs a good deal of work from the muscles of the trunk, and unless they are in working trim, your back may be strained. The secret is foot position, so that every action is a use of balanced body weight. Where space is too cramped, you may do better by getting down on your hands and knees.

Kneeling is a very sensible posture for many jobs in the garden. For a gardener who can neither stoop nor kneel nor squat, raised borders for flowers or a greenhouse with shelves would be possible outlets.

Digging is a traditional back-breaker for those untrained to it. Do not attempt to dig too much at one time. Stand over the job and try not to overload the fork or spade.

The wheelbarrow puts considerable stress on the spine because it has to be lifted and at the same time pushed; this is all very well if the ground is hard and level, but a great effort when the ground is soft and steep or uneven. If you need to make use of a wheelbarrow, choose one that takes the load well forward over the wheel; then, when you load it, make sure to place the load over the wheel so that the lifting effort needed is small. Be sure to lift the barrow correctly; stand between the shafts, bending at the hips and knees to reach the handles, then straighten at the hips and knees, lean forward with your body weight, and move off. It is better to make two journeys with small loads than to struggle with one.

Mowing the lawn

Lawnmowers, especially mechanical ones, are heavy, yet have to be heaved backwards, humped over lawn edges and in and out of sheds. Pushed mowers are the lightest and comparatively easy to manoeuvre. When using a push mower, wear boots or shoes with a good grip and use your body weight to help the movements.

Of the powered mowers, the lightest are those with electric motors which run off the mains, followed by those with petrol engines; the heaviest, weighing nearly 45kg, are electric mowers which run off accumulators. Cylinder mowers are on the whole heavier than rotary mowers, but, being more compact, are easier to manoeuvre. Rotary mowers are handy for rough grass but there the effort of manoeuvring is far greater, particularly if the mower has small wheels. Modern hover mowers are relatively light and effective while at the same time quite easy to manoeuvre.

Many people empty the grass box into a wheelbarrow, but unless you have an ergonomically satisfactory barrow or cart, it may be easier to empty the grass box on to a sheet with handles at the corners which is easy to pull across the lawn to the compost heap. Alternatively, if your back is suspect and you do not mind, leave the grass cuttings on the lawn instead of collecting them in the box.

With mowing, as with all gardening and other heavy work, the rule is not to do too much at a time. Plan all the work so that you can divide it into many short sessions, rather than a few long ones, and allow plenty of time to do the work. If working alongside somebody else, do not feel that you have to keep up;

work at your own pace. If your back starts hurting, do not struggle on to finish because the weather is right or you are going away tomorrow – stop.

Driving a car

Driving is an activity which gives a lot of people backache, even if they are otherwise free of back trouble. The problem is basically that you drive in a flexed posture, and the effects are made much worse by any deficiencies in the design and construction of the seat itself. Most car seats give poor lumbar support, and no lateral thigh support.

Adjust the car seat and angle of the back rest so that the pedals and the gear lever and steering wheel can be comfortably reached. In most cars, the runners of the seat can be moved so that you have more backward and forward positions. Before you make alterations to your driving seat, check that this will not interfere with your vision and control.

First the seat, then the car

Anybody buying a new car should ensure that the seat is adjustable, but should also try and have an opportunity of driving someone else's car of the same make for at least half an hour, failing which, ask the vendor for a test drive or hire a car for a day. If this is not possible, travelling as a front-seat passenger in the car may give some idea as to whether the seat of that particular make is suitable for a person with back problems. It is not possible to form a true impression by sitting in a stationary vehicle. When trying out a new car seat, it takes about half an hour of continuous driving to be able to predict how comfortable it will be on a long journey.

A car's seat should never be so springy that you bounce more than it does, and the padding should give lateral support to prevent your being thrown sideways on cornering, otherwise the spine is unsupported. If there is not enough lumbar support, use a cushion or anything that gives support in the small of the back. However, it is better not to use an inflatable cushion: this will aggravate the problem of lack of sideways control, because on cornering and pressing on pedals, air in the cushion may move to the 'wrong' side and this will tend to force the body into an even worse lateral displacement.

Car accessory shops sell numerous aids to seat comfort. Anything that supports your lower back and prevents it from flexing, or gives added sideways support, may help. Wooden bead mats that hang on the back of the seat are found helpful by some people. A back rest can be individually moulded to fit you in any seat, but you must be able to fix it securely to the car seat – ask the supplier about this. Remember, however, that anything inserted for seat comfort occupies space and reduces its effective length.

Driving
Backache from car driving is partly a postural stress but some of it comes from the movements of the car transmitted to the driver.

While driving, you scarcely change your position and your range of movements is restricted by the position of the hand and foot controls. Try to be relaxed while driving. To help prevent tenseness and stiffness in the neck, whenever you have to stop – for instance, at lights or in traffic jams – move your neck about a bit: shrug your shoulders a few times, raising them as high as possible towards your ears and then suddenly drop them.

It helps on a long journey to stop and take a little exercise at frequent intervals. Taking a short walk, even just around the car, provides a change of position, and therefore movement of the back. When stopping for petrol, always get out of the car.

Getting in and out
When climbing out of a car, get used to swivelling your whole body towards the door, then slide your feet on to the ground together, and stand up. Do not twist round to pick up parcels from the back seat.

A four-door car makes life with small children much easier on the back than a two-door car. If you have the latter, get into the rear with the child, and then strap him or her into the seat.

Luggage in the car
When travelling by car, loading it can be a problem. Many car boots have a high sill to hump the luggage over, and this imposes

a major stress, especially when having to duck under the lid of the boot. If the floor of the boot is lower than the edge of the boot opening, limit the weight of individual pieces of luggage so that they can be easily swung up to rest on the sill of the boot, then lowered with one hand while you support yourself with the other hand. Keep the floor of the boot clear of clutter so that the suitcases can easily be pushed into position. Avoid trying to push things sideways. If you can, move your feet so that you pull things into place rather than having to twist your body to heave them about.

Air travel

Airline seats vary in comfort according to the price. Economy-class seats are designed to be particularly mean with elbow and leg room, but on long journeys even the more expensive seats can leave you feeling stiff. Get up and walk about now and again if you possibly can.

Sleeping in your seat has to be done in one position – leaning back – and that is usually a sure way to a stiff neck. The inadequate little cushions handed out by the airlines on long-distance flights are not much help: placed behind the neck, they keep sliding out. Most airport shops and luggage shops sell U-shaped inflatable cushions which support the neck quite efficiently, and the airline's cushion can go in the small of your back.

Carrying luggage

Pack and unpack a suitcase downstairs to avoid having to lug it down or up the stairs when it is full and heavy.

A shoulder bag, such as an airline carry-on bag or a rucksack, is better than a hand-held bag, provided this does not lead to uneven posture on one side; try putting the strap diagonally across your body rather than over one shoulder, or carry two evenly-loaded bags, one in each hand.

Suitcases and holdalls can be troublesome to someone liable to back pain. The logical solution to carrying luggage is to divide the load into three: in a rucksack over your shoulders, and one small case in each hand.

A suitcase with its own wheels can take much of the lifting out of moving luggage. Make sure that the handle is at a comfortable height, that the suitcase comes with a strap to pull it along, otherwise trying to wheel a small suitcase with castors underneath would mean walking with an awkwardly twisted spine.

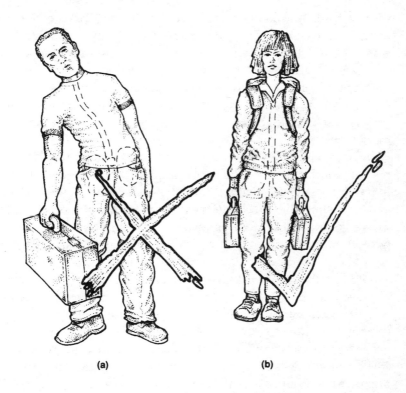

(a)   (b)

(a) Don't carry all your luggage in one big suitcase. The dotted line shows how it affects the spine and pelvis

(b) Better for the spine to spread the load, with a smaller suitcase in each hand and a rucksack on the back

CHAPTER 16

EXERCISE

IT is a truth universally acknowledged that regular exercise is good for the health. The huge interest that people in Western countries have been showing in their own health in recent years has been accompanied by growing participation in many forms of activity. There are many exercise programmes and schemes to be found, so it is as well to make sure before embarking on any for the first time that they are safe and effective, with properly trained tutors.

Many people who take up sports or games do not follow a regular routine, and risk injuring their health rather than improving it. To be effective and safe, exercise must be regular, and a set time should be allocated for it each day. You should strictly follow a graduated programme of exercises, and as far as possible make sure that you are building up muscular strength equally on both sides of the vertebral column.

The fact that a wide spectrum of problems and disorders are improved by a regular exercise regime is often overlooked. Regular exercise helps prevent conditions like heart disease, thinning of bones (osteoporosis), high blood pressure and possibly even a stroke. Even frail, older people may benefit from an exercise routine. The positive, psychological effects are just as important as the physical benefits. Recreational exercise allows people to mix with others who may otherwise be isolated and even lonely. In addition, regular exercise has been shown to reduce anxiety levels as well as relieving stress. There is also good scientific evidence to suggest that regular exercise helps improve the quality of sleep. The mood-enhancing effect after a work out has been attributed (though by no means proven) to the release of natural morphine-like compounds within the body. However, don't get too carried away as there are situations when it is advisable not to exercise, for example during an illness such as a viral infection or a fever. Also, embarking on a work-out shortly after a heavy meal is not wise.

Sports and athletics

Each sporting and athletic activity has its own techniques, which must be learned and practised, for preventing damage to joints, ligaments and muscles. Even professional sportsmen, athletes and gymnasts, who train constantly, quite often suffer from strains and sprains, and anybody who goes in for such activities without adequate training and preparation is very likely to suffer for it.

If you go in for sport as relaxation from work, you should be restrained in your ambition, and not be so competitive that you disregard your health and safety.

One golden rule for sport which should always be followed is: warm up before you start. Gymnasts and ballet dancers always start with some gentle exercises designed to warm up joints and muscles which have not been used for a while. They know that to start work cold is to invite injury. Warm-up exercises should: stretch the postural muscles; loosen and stretch all the leg joints and foot joints; stretch the arm and hand joints. If you intend to be involved in sport, it is important to train and play regularly, otherwise you risk injury. Do not train or play when you are injured. In attempting to protect one injury you may precipitate another; for example, prolonged limping may aggravate or initiate a back problem.

Which sport?

No sport is good or bad in itself; what counts is how you go about it. But for anyone with back trouble (past or present) some are not advisable, such as rugby, parachuting and trampolining.

Walking

Both walking and running can be valuable in helping to prevent obesity, and are both natural activities which, if done with proper

131

care, make a demand on the postural muscles which may help to prevent back problems. Walking is increasingly the preferred alternative to jogging.

If you do run or jog, it is important to reduce the jarring effect which is transmitted to the back if poorly cushioned, badly designed (this usually means cheap) shoes are worn. Old training shoes may also cause trouble because even though the sole is not worn out, the midsole has lost its cushioning powers.

Always wear comfortable, well-fitting shoes. Lace-up styles with thick light soles or trainers are ideal. Some people find it useful to add a pair of shock-absorbing insoles or heel pads, obtainable from larger chemists or sports shops.

When walking, walk tall, keep your tummy tucked in and let your arms swing. Start with short walks and gradually increase the distance. As walking becomes easier, increase your speed and stride.

Walking around the shops, dodging people, stopping to look in shop windows and standing at check-outs does not constitute walking as a helpful exercise. In fact, many people who do not otherwise have backache find that an afternoon's shopping can cause it. A real walk should be part of your regular routine: around the block or the nearest park to start with and gradually, as your walking fitness improves, you will be able to go further afield.

Swimming

Swimming provides the body with good all-round exercise. It encourages mobility and, without putting undue strain on the spine, promotes muscle strength. It is valuable for people with back problems: the water provides support, and the exercise can be undertaken without stressing the spinal column. The buoyancy of the water minimises the effects of body weight, making it easier to move.

The most effective strokes are front crawl and back-stroke which give the whole body regular and rhythmic movement. If you swim breast-stroke, try not to keep your head out of the water all the time, as this extended position can put a strain on your neck. Try wearing goggles and learn to breathe out with your face under water. In this way the head is kept in line with

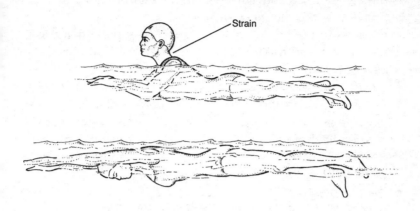

Strain

the body and the neck stress minimised. There are also exercises other than swimming that can be done in the water which may also benefit the back, for example, aqua aerobics in classes at health clubs and swimming pools. As well as being good for your back, it is fun.

Exercising at home

Exercises for the back are intended to strengthen and improve the postural regulating powers of the spinal muscles. The vertebral joints do not need to be exercised because the spine is never at rest, even when you are in bed. Stiffness in these joints can be helped by exercise only if it is due to weakness in the muscles and ligaments; it can be helped by gently working the muscles. But when there is stiffness as a result of a disc prolapse, misaligned facet joints or curvature, exercises can do harm rather than good.

Exercises that do not help a bad back
There are some kinds of exercises which should be positively avoided when you are recovering from back pain, and done with caution at all times:

133

- bending forwards is supposed to strengthen the abdominal muscles, but is not advisable where the pressure can push a disc protrusion into the spinal canal
- exercises to stretch the spine are given by some instructors to reduce disc protrusion and strengthen back muscles, but excessive bending backwards can damage the facet joints
- bending sideways can be beneficial in moderation, but always involves some rotation of each vertebra, so that the exercise needs to be done slowly, carefully and over a short range
- rotation has been thought to mobilise stiff joints, but excessive rotation is harmful: since the immobile joints cannot be moved, the mobile ones will be overstrained
- toe touching used to be one of the classic exercises for fitness but to touch your toes while standing (or while sitting) with legs straight and feet apart is likely to do more harm than good, particularly if you use the opposite hand, so adding a twisting motion
- double leg raising, often recommended as an abdominal strengthening exercise, can be positively harmful because it puts considerable strain on the lower back. During this exercise the hip muscles have to do most of the work and as they are attached to the lower lumbar vertebrae and the pelvis, the abdominal muscles are called upon to stabilise the pelvis while the legs are lifted. The weight of straight legs makes it too difficult for the abdominal muscles to continue to hold the pelvis, which tilts forward. This causes the lumbar spine to hollow as the spinal joints are pulled forward, putting considerable strain on them
- lifting both legs up straight, or sitting up from lying with a straight back, are two exercises which should not be carried out except by someone exceptionally fit and well muscled.

Exercises for the back

Movement is necessary for the maintenance of a healthy spine. Regular physical activity helps to ensure that the joints remain mobile and the muscles strong. A stiff spine with weak supporting muscles cannot cope with the additional stress that might be imposed on it by some unaccustomed position or sudden awkward movement.

It is therefore extremely important if you have a back problem, or have had one in the past, to ensure that your spine is as mobile as possible and supported by strong muscles.

You should not carry out any exercise in a way that causes pain which continues after the exercise is finished. However, if your spine is very stiff, you may feel some discomfort while stretching. As long as this discomfort goes when you stop the exercise, it is likely to be helping to restore your range of movement and will become easier on subsequent occasions. If the discomfort persists, omit that exercise.

Why does exercise help?

If the back is diseased, some of the muscles that work with the spinal column will weaken, in the same way that the muscle bulk in a limb will start to wither if the limb is injured or paralysed and not moved properly. A regular exercise routine designed for back sufferers will improve the strength and bulk of the muscles attached to the spinal column, restoring their ability to control the normal maintenance of spinal posture. In addition it will off-load the extra strain placed on the bones and joints which have had to take over some of the affected muscle's role.

An exercise regime will also have a positive effect on the person's state of mind and attitude. Many people with backache, either with an acute attack or a chronic problem, may lose their confidence to the extent that they over-protect their back. A carefully-put-together exercise routine, preferably under the guidance of an experienced and qualified instructor, can work wonders, restoring the sufferer's confidence in his or her back, when he or she would otherwise be fearful to use it.

Choosing a class

The actual form of the exercise, be it aerobics, step or a more sedate form of exercise, is not particularly relevant. It is more important to choose a class that runs at a pace that you can keep up with. There is no point in enrolling in a class for very fit people when you are unfit with a back problem; your condition may well end up being worse than when you started. Make sure the teacher is experienced and has had some form of formal training. The class should have room to accommodate all the participants easily, with reasonable room to spare. Always remember to limber up slowly if you are working out to music, making sure you can hear the teacher's instructions above the level of the music. Most importantly, don't be frightened to ask for advice: a good teacher will be pleased to answer your questions about the class.

CHAPTER **17**

MYTHS AND MYSTERIES: FACT AND FICTION

Backache is a major problem

In 1993, 150 million working days were lost through backache in Britain: 50 million were due to sufferers spending short periods of time away from work, and 100 million because people left their employment altogether, claiming sickness and invalidity benefits. Statistics vary dramatically, depending on what exactly is being measured, and it is possible that even this total of 150 million is an underestimate. Despite these staggering statistics, many people are ashamed to admit that they are suffering from back pain, fearing that colleagues may believe them to be work-shy or even that they are wrongly taking sick leave.

The more the field of backache is looked into, the more obvious it becomes that there are many large gaps in what is known about it. It is therefore not surprising that many misconceptions have evolved. Some popular myths associated with backache follow:

I've been struck down with backache for the first time and I'm in terrible pain. I think I ought to see the doctor but I might not be able to get an appointment straight away, and he or she will probably only send me away with painkillers. You are not alone in thinking that a visit to the doctor, which may well involve a wait, is inconvenient and perhaps unnecessary. In fact, it is thought that less than half of those who have an episode of backache will consult their GP.

It is indeed probable that your backache is not serious and that you will be sent away with painkillers and told to rest for a few days. However, it might be that your pain is caused by something more serious than, for example, straightforward backache, so it is important that a diagnosis is made. A visit is free, and if you do not usually pay for a prescription, all further treatment will be free.

It may be that you would prefer to visit a therapist, for example, an osteopath or chiropractor, instead. These practitioners have gained in stature in the public eye over the last few years and now play an important role in the treatment and prevention of backache. People with back pain who were treated by a chiropractor received more benefit than those receiving hospital out-patient treatment.

Will I have to have an X-ray to find out what is wrong with my back? An X-ray is not always needed; many episodes of backache are caused by soft tissues such as muscles and discs, not by bone problems. Soft tissues do not tend to show up very well on an X-ray, and the results are rarely significant enough to affect the direct management of a problem. Changes that do show up often correlate poorly with the symptoms and signs of backache. X-rays tend to be more helpful if the symptoms are prolonged or if something more serious is suspected.

There are times when an X-ray should be avoided: for example, a woman who is either trying to conceive or is pregnant should avoid having one of her pelvis, as this would expose the unborn baby to radiation, putting it at risk. However, there will be circumstances when an X-ray cannot be avoided, for example if a serious disease is suspected.

I am 40 years old and have pain in my lower back and buttocks. There is no reason that I can think of that it should have happened; I'm worried that something serious is causing it. Characteristically, if a person is between the ages of 20 and 50 and the pain is in the lower back, buttocks or even thighs, the condition is more likely to be simple backache. It can occur for no apparent reason or as a direct result of a particular activity. Apart from feeling pain, the sufferer will otherwise feel well. The outlook is positive as about 90 per cent of episodes are likely to recover within about six weeks, though it can recur at a later date. The names that are usually given to this type of pain are lumbago, or mechanical backache.

As well as backache, I have pins and needles. The pain sometimes travels down just one leg. What could be causing this? This could be nerve-root pain; it is more of a problem than simple backache because the nerve is impinged upon at some point near its exit from the spinal canal. As well as pins and needles some sufferers also experience numbness. About 50 per cent of sufferers recover from an episode of nerve-root pain in about six weeks. If the disturbance follows the course of the sciatic nerve, it is true sciatica (the word sciatica is often wrongly used to describe a general backache).

I've got backache and I'm terribly worried that it might be cancer. This is unlikely, as cancer is an uncommon cause of backache. Do not be alarmed if your doctor suggests that you have an isotope bone-scan or a blood test; it is important that cancer is eliminated from the possible causes of your pain.

Cancer can spread from an internal organ to the spine. Breast cancer in women and prostate cancer in men can be responsible for painful secondaries in the spine, although many other forms of malignancy can cause it, for example lung cancer in both men and women can affect the bony spinal column.

Sometimes backache can be the only symptom of a malignancy, and occasionally the primary malignancy is not identifiable. Significant symptoms to look out for include: constant and continuous backache, general recent ill health and perhaps recent weight loss. An X-ray, blood tests or even an isotope bone-scan will be needed to confirm the diagnosis. A tumour deposit may show up as a 'hot spot' on an isotope scan.

What is a collapsed vertebra? A collapsed vertebra can occur after a fall, spontaneously or after minimal trauma. Even if there is only a mild deformity of the affected vertebra, back pain may persist for some time after the incident, perhaps for up to two years. Occasionally it can be a life-long problem with on-going flare-ups.

Other common causes are osteoporosis or a tumour deposit. Both diseases weaken the structure of the vertebra, ultimately allowing it to collapse. Often there is little in the way of treatment apart from painkillers, though if a tumour is causing the pain, symptomatic treatment may be offered, using radiotherapy.

Having had backache for a long time, I have tried many different therapies and have been given a lot of advice, sometimes conflicting. Are there guidelines for doctors to follow about how they should deal with it? Doctors and other health professionals always like to adapt proven research results to everyday practice. Over the last few years, guidelines and information for the management of both common and uncommon conditions have appeared to try to help doctors to work in a more uniform way; backache is no exception. In 1994, a clinical standards advisory group, which acts as an independent source of expert advice to the British government, was commissioned to look at many aspects of back care in the NHS. The report called *Clinical Standards Advisory Group, Back Pain* (available from most HMSO bookshops) made some interesting and helpful suggestions for doctors in the management of backache. However, research conducted a couple of years later showed that the management of back pain by family doctors did not always follow the guidelines. The suggestions may have looked useful on paper, but perhaps did not translate well into everyday practice.

I am suffering from severe back pain and I'm terribly worried that I will become a cripple. This is very rare, but it can happen. The vast majority of people can be reassured that they will not end up in a wheelchair.

I have heard that pain is simply a warning sign and that as long as I stop the activity that caused it, my back will be all right. Pain sometimes acts as a warning sign but only when it is acute; it is a short-term problem, and the result is that you stop the activity that you were doing, thereby preventing further injury. The pain actually restricts movement in the damaged area, giving it time to heal.

Chronic pain on the other hand may be as painful as an acute episode but it lasts much longer; because of this, it loses the role of an early-warning system and protector of an injured area. Ongoing pain can be extremely wearing, but even if the cause cannot be treated, the pain itself can. Chronic pain can be classified as a disorder in itself and can lead to, for example, a depressive illness, but this is potentially treatable.

I've had backache for a long time, and the doctors can't do any more for me. Will I now just have to grin and bear the pain? No, you won't. Medical science still has much to offer back-pain sufferers despite the fact that the underlying cause cannot be cured or precisely understood. Better understanding of how to control pain has allowed many people to have a reasonable quality of life. Pain clinics are available in most hospitals and although some of them have long waiting lists, it is well worth finding out, perhaps from your GP, what facilities are available in your area.

I've tried every treatment for my back pain, and I'm really worried that the only option open to me now is an operation. Surgery will benefit only a few backache sufferers, and with no guarantee of success. Unless it is an emergency, think carefully about the pros and cons of having an operation. Always ask questions about success rates, possible risks and the time taken to recover. It might be useful to speak to physiotherapists and occupational therapists who routinely look after post-operative patients. Most people are relieved to hear that they do not need an operation, though a few, who were hoping that it would cure them, are disappointed to hear that they will not benefit from surgery.

My back pain has gone on for a long time and I'm embarrassed about repeatedly going back to my doctor. Many people are reluctant to keep visiting the doctor, particularly if they feel that the problem cannot be cured. Doctors have been criticised for not listening to their patients, and it could be that they are not exploring your feelings properly. If this is the case, be direct with your questions, and if you don't get satisfactory answers, seek another opinion in the practice or consider changing your doctor.

You may feel, however, that complementary therapists could offer you better, alternative treatment to traditional medicine. Discussing your condition with a therapist such as a chiropractor, osteopath or acupuncturist may help you to understand your problem, even if it cannot be cured.

I've been told that I have spondylolysis, but I have also seen the term spondylosis – are they two different conditions? Yes, they are, and it is very easy to mix them up. However, the symptoms are very different. Spondylolysis is a break in the structure of a vertebra, often associated with spondylolisthesis, whereas spondylosis is an abnormally fixed and immobile vertebral joint.

There are two common varieties of spondylosis, affecting the neck and the lower back; these are called cervical and lumbar spondylosis respectively. These are commonly found in people over 40. Spondylosis is also often considered together with osteoarthritis and grouped with it as a degenerative disorder.

Cervical spondylosis is a common condition often causing pain across the back of the neck, shoulders and radiating down one or both arms. It can be difficult, diagnostically, to separate this problem from shoulder abnormalities such as arthritis or a frozen shoulder. The usual treatment consists of painkillers or anti-inflammatory drugs and possibly a neck collar for a short period. The symptoms of lumbar spondylosis are similar to degenerative joint problems: loss of movement and pain after movement. The treatment is similar to that for cervical spondylosis, and a corset should be used judiciously, if at all.

I have had an episode of backache and have been told that it is fine for me to go back to work as my job is sedentary. This is not necessarily the right advice. A large number of people, despite being well motivated and willing to do any job, find that they cannot cope with a sedentary job. For example, office work can place quite a strain on the back, making it potentially intolerable for the back sufferer. Typing and a badly organised desk in particular may make it worse.

My backache has continued for quite some time. Treatment won't do me any harm, so I may as well try something. I have nothing to lose. Most therapies will have some sort of side-effect and may even do more harm than good. No matter how innocuous or high-tech the treatment seems to be, always ask about potential side-effects and weigh them up against the chances of a successful outcome. There is an argument in certain situations that to do nothing is a sensible option.

I have been told that my disc has slipped. Will it be easy to put back in place? Slipped discs are often blamed for all sorts of back problems but in fact they do not and cannot slip. This misconception leads people to believe that if the disc has slipped, it can be put back in place easily. This is far from the truth. 'Slipped disc' is, in fact, a term used when the disc has bulged and impinges on a nerve as a result.

What can I do to protect my spine? Once your back is damaged it is unlikely that it will ever be restored to its original state. Although surgery can help occasionally, it will not put right all the damage. The answer is to make sure that you keep your back in good shape, thereby preventing injury in the first place. Procedures like lifting properly and avoiding sitting in one position for too long are simple rules to try to follow. Remember: it is better to keep your back moving than keeping still. These rules also apply to preventing a recurrence of the injury.

I would like to visit an osteopath as I feel that my doctor cannot offer me any further treatment, but I am worried that he or she will disapprove. This is unlikely. There are a some reasons why you might not want to tell your doctor that you are going to visit another therapist: you may feel that he or she has not given you the kind of support and understanding that you need; the doctor may not believe in the effectiveness of your chosen alternative treatment. Only a very small minority of doctors may be perturbed, believing that your choosing to visit another practitioner means that they have not looked after you properly. More often it is the case that GPs actively encourage their patients to visit other therapists. It is probably best to inform your doctor of all the treatment you are having or intend to have, if only to note this on your medical records. If for whatever reason you do not want to tell your GP that you are going to see an osteopath, for example, you do not have to. You do not need to be referred to, for example, an osteopath, acupuncturist or chiropractor – you can contact them directly, although it is likely that you will have to pay a fee.

I have a prolapsed disc and my doctor has told me that I should stay in bed for a maximum of three days, but I always understood that as much bed rest as possible is the best cure. In the past it was thought that absolute bed rest was the best cure for a bad back, and there are people who still think that this is the case. However, this idea has now been disregarded. A few days' bed rest is fine (for more than one to three days) when the pain first strikes. After that, it is best to keep moving even if there is an initial increase in pain. Lack of movement can make the joints and muscles stiff, and gentle exercise can help to strengthen them.

People going through litigation never recover from backache. There seems to be a widespread belief that people involved in litigation with a back problem or whiplash injury are unlikely to recover so as to justify their case. This is often an unfair accusation – many people involved in legal tussles have sustained quite genuine injuries.

GLOSSARY

Adhesions   Sticking together of tissues due to inflammation

Ankylosing spondylitis   An inflammatory disease of unknown origin, which may affect the mobility of the spine

Annulus fibrosus   Outer casing of intervertebral disc

Apophyseal joint   Facet joint

Arachnoiditis   An inflammation of the arachnoid mater membrane, causing it to thicken, and so impede the movement of nerve roots inside the dural sleeves

Arachnoid mater   See *dural tube*

Arthritis   Inflammation of the joints

Atlas *and* axis   The first two cervical vertebrae: the atlas supports the head and, in turn, is supported by the axis; together they permit nodding, side flexion and rotation of the head

Cauda equina   The bundle of lumbar and sacral nerve roots at the end of the spinal cord (Latin – horse's tail)

Cervical   Relating to the neck (Latin – cervix)

Chronic   Of long duration

Coccyx   Termination of the base of the spine; a vestigial tail, consisting of four tiny fused vertebrae

Disc, intervertebral disc   One of the 23 shock-absorbing pads lying between adjacent pairs of vertebral bodies; each consists of a tough, fibrous outer casing (the annulus fibrosus) enclosing a gel-like core (the nucleus pulposus)

Dislocation   Condition of a joint in which the bones become disconnected from each other

Dorsal   An alternative name for the thoracic part of the spine (Latin – dorsum, the back)

Dural sleeves   The sheaths protecting the nerve roots as they branch off from the spinal cord

Dural tube   The sheath of the spinal cord; it consists of three membranes: the innermost one is the pia mater; this is enclosed in the arachnoid mater; the toughest outermost one is the dura mater

Dura mater   See *dural tube*

Epidural root fibrosis   Abnormal increase of fibrous tissue round a nerve root, resulting from inflammation of the dural sleeve

Extensor   Muscle that extends or straightens out a part of the body

Facet joint   Also known as apophyseal joint. The joint formed by the faceted surfaces of the bones which are covered with cartilage and slide over each other inside a fibrous capsule lined with synovial membrane and lubricated with synovial fluid. This type of joint is found between the processes of adjacent vertebrae

Fascia   Thin sheet of connective tissue covering a muscle

Fibrin   Protein which forms when blood clots when tissues are injured; it is the body's natural repair material. Adhesions form when the excess fibrin from an injured membrane fastens it to another tissue

Fibrositis   Inflammation of connective tissue fibres: term is used to denote intermittent localised pain in small areas of muscles or ligaments, possibly resulting from tension or bad posture

Foramen (*plural:*** foramina)**   Gap between the pedicles of adjacent vertebrae, through which the nerve roots emerge as they branch out from the spinal cord

Kyphosis   Convex curvature of the spine, which occurs naturally in the thoracic spine and in the region where the sacrum joins the coccyx; if it is excessive, or is present elsewhere in the spine, it is a deformity. See also *lordosis*

Lamina (*plural:*** laminae)**   A part of the neural arch, lying between the spinous process and the pedicle

Lesion Any unfavourable change in the functioning or texture of organs and tissues; used by some doctors to mean a change assumed to be the cause of pain

Ligament Band of fibrous tissue binding the bones of a joint; it controls the range of movement by allowing it only in certain directions

Lordosis A concave curvature of the spine, which occurs naturally in the cervical and the lumbar spine; if it is excessive or occurs elsewhere in the spine, it is a deformity. See also *kyphosis*

Lumbago Imprecise term meaning pain in the lumbar region: low back pain

Lumbar Relating to the area of the back between the thoracic spine and the sacrum (Latin – lumbum, the loin)

Myelography X-ray visualisation (using radio-opaque dye) of the space inside the spinal canal surrounding the spinal cord and nerve roots

Nerve root The origin of a nerve as it leaves the spinal cord; one of a pair of bands of nervous tissue branching out of the spinal cord at the level of each vertebra, and passing outwards through a foramen

Neural arch The ring of bone at the back of each vertebra; it is made up of the following projections: two pedicles, two transverse processes, two superior and two inferior articular processes and the spinous process

Nucleus pulposus The gel-like core of an intervertebral disc

Osteoarthritis See *osteoarthrosis*

Osteoarthrosis Degeneration of joints, generally accompanied by the thickening of bone; also called osteoarthritis, but it is not an inflammatory condition

Osteomalacia Bone disease in which vitamin D deficiency in adults causes loss of calcium from, and softening of, the bones

Osteophyte Bony outgrowth of spur forming on a bone

Osteophytosis The proliferation of osteophytes at more than one site, usually accompanied by general thickening of bone

Osteoporosis Bone disease characterised by loss of bone substance, thus making bones more easily fractured

Paget's disease Bone disease in which bones become thicker, but also softer, tending to deform

Pedicle Part of the neural arch; each neural arch has two pedicles

Pia mater See *dural tube*

Prolapse In the case of an intervertebral disc, this means the rupture of the disc's outer casing, and the leaking out of part of the nucleus through the rupture

Reflex Involuntary reaction of the muscles to some stimulus which does not rise to the level of consciousness; reflex actions, such as jerking the hand away when touching a hot object, are controlled by the nerves of the spinal cord

Retrolisthesis A backwards displacement of one or more vertebrae

Rheumatism Not a disease, but a vague term used for aches and pains in muscles and joints

Rheumatoid arthritis Inflammatory disease, which may be progressive, of the synovial joints in any part of the body

Sacroiliac joint Joint occurring between each side of the sacrum and the adjoining part of the pelvis called the ilium

Sacrum Curved, wedge-shaped bone, consisting of five fused vertebrae, at the lower end of the spine, between the two halves of the pelvis

Sciatica Not a disease, but the name given to a sharp pain in the area of distribution of the sciatic nerve – that is, along the back of the thigh and down the whole leg; sciatic pain can arise when a disorder of the lumbar spine causes pressure on a nerve root

Scoliosis A sideways curvature of the spine. A structural scoliosis may be a congenital deformity; a postural scoliosis occurs when the spine is bent to reduce pressure on a compressed nerve root and so lessen the pain

Slipped disc A misnomer for a prolapsed disc; intervertebral discs do not slip

Spasm; muscular spasm An involuntary muscular response to injury; the muscles automatically tighten round the site, and this serves to prevent movement of the painful tissues; spasm occurs as a result of over-excitation or stimulation of muscle cells by nerve impulses

Spinal canal   The conduit formed by the neural arches and bodies of the vertebrae through which the spinal cord passes

Spinal cord   A continuation of the brain along the spinal canal, in the form of a long band of nervous tissue, inside the dural tube; it is the main highway of the nervous system, conveying information to and from the brain

Spondylitis   Inflammation of vertebrae

Spondylolisthesis   A deformity of the spine in which a vertebra slips forward on the one below, so that the whole of the spine above it is also displaced

Spondylolysis   Fracture of the neural arch which may be the cause of spondylolisthesis

Spondylosis   Osteoarthritis of the facet joints together with degeneration of discs; the bone thickening may result in encroachment into the spinal canal

Stenosis   Narrowing of some passage or canal in the body. Lateral stenosis occurs when for some reason the width of a foramen is restricted, compressing the nerve root inside it; central canal stenosis occurs when the spinal cord is compressed by some reduction in the width of the spinal canal

Subluxation   When the bones in a joint are displaced but not completely dislocated

Synovial joint   Joint enclosed in a fibrous capsule lined with the synovial membrane

Synovium (synovial membrane)   Moist membrane lining the capsule which encloses a synovial joint (for example a facet joint); it is lubricated with synovial fluid

Tendon   Tough fibrous elongation of a muscle, serving to attach it to a bone

Thoracic   Relating to the chest (Latin – thorax)

Vertebra (*plural* vertebrae)   One of the 24 bones, stacked on top of each other and separated by discs, which, together with the sacrum and the coccyx, make up the spinal column

ADDRESSES

Acupuncture Association of
Chartered Physiotherapists
Hilltop
Benjamin Road
High Wycombe
Buckinghamshire HP13 6SR
(01494) 451295

Arthritis and Rheumatism
Council
PO Box 177
Chesterfield
Derbyshire S41 7TQ
(01246) 558033

British Acupuncture
Association
34 Alderney Street
London SW1V 4EU
0171-834 1012

British Acupuncture Council
Park House
206 Latimer Road
London W10 6RE
0181-964 0222

British Chiropractic
Association
29 Whitley Street
Reading
Berkshire RG2 0EG
(01734) 757557

British College of
Naturopathy and Osteopathy
Frazer House
6 Netherhall Gardens
London NW3 5RR
0171-435 6464

British Medical Acupuncture
Society
Newton House
Newton Lane
Whitley
Warrington
Cheshire WA4 4JA
(01925) 730727

British Osteopathic
Association
8–10 Boston Place
London NW1 6QH
0171-262 5250

British School of Osteopathy
1/4 Suffolk Street
London SW1Y 4HG
0171-930 9254

Chartered Society of
Physiotherapy
14 Bedford Row
London WC1R 4ED
0171-242 1941

The Disabled Living
Foundation
380-4 Harrow Road
London W9 2HU
0171-289 6111

European School of
Osteopathy
104 Tonbridge Road
Maidstone
Kent ME16 8SL
(01622) 671558

The Feldenkrais Guild
PO Box 370
London N10 3XA

The General Council and
Register of Naturopaths
(GCRN)
Goswell House
2 Goswell Road
Street
Somerset BA16 0JG
(01458) 840072

General Council and Register
of Osteopaths (GCRO)
56 London Street
Reading
Berkshire RG1 4SQ
(01734) 576585

Institute of Complementary
Medicine
PO Box 194
London SE16 1QZ

London College of
Osteopathic Medicine
(See British Osteopathic
Association)

National Ankylosing
Spondylitis Society
5 Grosvenor Crescent
London SW1X 7ER
0171-235 9585

The National Back Pain
Association
16 Elmtree Road
Teddington
Middlesex TW11 8ST
0181-977 5474

Osteopathic Information
Service
PO Box 2074
Reading
Berkshire RG1 4YR
(01734) 512051

Scoliosis Association UK
325 Latimer Road
London W10
0181-964 5343

Pain Concern UK
PO Box 318
Canterbury
Kent CT2 0DG
(01227) 712183

Shiatsu Society
c/o 5 Foxcote
Wokingham
Berkshire RG11 3PG
(01483) 860771

Society of Teachers of the
Alexander Technique (STAT)
20 London House
266 Fulham Road
London SW10 9EL
0171-351 0828

Spinal Injuries Association
76 St James's Lane
London N10 3DF
(Counselling line 0181-883
4296, Mon–Fri, 2–5pm)

Other useful addresses

Arthritis Care
18 Stephenson Way
London NW1 2HD
0171-916 1500

British Massage Therapy
Council
Greenbank House
65a Adelphi Street
Preston
Lancashire PR1 7BH
(01772) 881063

British Reflexology
Association
Monks Orchard
Whitbourne
Worcestershire WR6 5RB
(01886) 21207

The International Federation
of Aromatherapy
Stamford House
2–4 Chiswick High Road
London W4 1TH

Organisation of Chartered
Physiotherapists in Private
Practice (OCPPP)
Suite 8, Weston Chambers
Weston Road
Southend on Sea
Essex SS1 1AT
(01702) 392124

Repetitive Strain Injury
Association
Chapel House
152 High Street
Yiewsley
West Drayton
Middlesex UB7 7BE
(01895) 431134 (Mon–Fri,
11.30am–4pm)

INDEX